Tips & Tricks from Eastern Europe

Nutrition & Exercise

Roxana P. Samson

Roxana P. Samson

Description:

This is a complete manual for weight loss, gain muscles and stay in shape forever. The book describes healthy nutrition and types of exercise. This is for both, a regular individual and a future competitor. Looking good does not relate to your age. Everything is information and desire. We need to know a correct way of doing exercise for no accidents and for progression. We need to know the right foods and combinations in order to help our body to recover from a toxic life. The book comprehends lots of details about nutrition, about aerobic and anaerobic exercise, details which will always stay as basic principles. When we wish to enhance our nourishment by using supplements, we must know the times and types we may ingest them and the reason. Otherwise, they are not effective and some of them trigger unwanted weight gain. If you are an individual hoping to compete one day, you have a chapter just for you, describing the last week preparation and other important details. This book may stay as a guide for the personal trainer. Every page of this work comprehends useful information and it will not waste your time.

Roxana P. Samson

Table of Contents

Chapter 1

Nutrition

1.1. Proteins

The proteins are the building blocks for muscular mass. Without eating protein, it will be hard for us to build muscles. Unfortunately, the protein in regular foods, comes together with fat. We should try to eat lean meats and not too many processed meats. Additionally, protein supports the immune system and protects the body against viruses and bacteria. We may take protein from different sources. It comes from meat, eggs, dairy, nuts, cereals and vegetables. It is important to know that not all the sources have the complete protein. In this case, our body has to form the complete protein which does not come as a whole from outside. That gives more work to do for our system but it comes as a natural process for the body itself and this is nothing to worry about.

The complete protein exists in meat, dairy and eggs. The protein coming from nuts and the majority of vegetables, it identifies as not a complete protein. Couple vegetables do contain the complete protein as soy and quinoa.

Complete protein means that it has all the main essential amino acids. Usually, there are 20 amino acids in total and 8 of them are essential. These numbers are little different when we read other materials. Certain studies show there are 23 amino acids in total and 9 essential amino acids. There is Histidine, an amino acid which is added to those 8 essential amino acids. Specialists found it as being essential for babies only, adults being able to synthesize it by themselves. The other 8 essential amino acids are: Isoleucine, Leucine, Valine, Lysine, Methionine, Phenylalanine, Threonine, Tryptophan. Here may be added 2 semi essential amino acids which are sometimes essential, too: Cysteine and Tyrosine. These amino acids are called essential because it is mandatory to introduce them into the diet for a good health. The others are not mandatory for the body, that is why they are called not essential. There are 11 not essential amino acids: Alanine, Arginine, Asparagine, Aspartic Acid, Cysteine, Glutamic Acid, Glutamine, Glycine, Tyrosine, Proline, Serine.

When a protein is not complete, as the protein from beans or rice, it does not have all the essential amino acids in its composition to be able to be absorbed in the body. Our system needs to find soon the rest of the essential amino acids to form the complete protein and use it as nutrition. These 8 essential amino acids cannot be produced by the body itself. We have to take them from the outside food. Our body has the ability to produce the not essential amino acids and it is not mandatory to take them from outside, from the food.

Sources of animal protein:
- fish, sea food, beef, chicken, turkey, duck, goat, lamb, pork, eggs, cheese, milk or even bear, deer and other special meats. All these above have the complete protein and they contain all the 8 essential amino acids.

Sources of vegetable protein:

- beans, peas, cereals, rice, quinoa (complete protein), seeds, nuts, soy (complete protein), etc.

Usually, the ones coming from vegetable sources have an incomplete protein, meaning the body need to combine them with other nutrients to form the complete protein. In order to do so, below there are few examples. Otherwise, let's hope our body will be smart enough to find by himself the necessary amino acids to combine.

Forming complete protein we may try:
- rice + beans (cereal + vegetable)
- rice + lentils (cereal + vegetable)
- hazelnuts/almonds/walnuts + beans (nuts + vegetable)
- whole wheat pasta + cheese (cereals + dairy)
- dairy + seeds
- vegetables + seeds

Rice and beans is the perfect combination to form the complete protein. Usually, 3 spoons of rice work with 1 spoon of beans. For vegetarians and not only, these are very good choices. But, when we want to build muscle mass, we do not need to consider these or other vegetables for protein counting. Even if they contain some proteins, the amount of protein per day has to be counted from the complete protein sources only.

Quinoa is a complete protein. It does not contain gluten as some of the cereals. It may successfully replace the cereals or the rice. Quinoa does not contain starch. The rice contains much amidine (starch) and helps to gain unwanted fat when eaten in high quantities. One cup of boiled quinoa has 8 grams of protein, almost twice fibers than other cereals and lots of minerals. Not to confuse Quinoa, the grains with chia, the seeds.

Chia seeds are also very nutritive for us, but they are different than quinoa. One spoon of chia is enough for a portion. It does not have a lot of proteins, but it is good to be mentioned for other nutritional reasons. Chia is very healthy to be consumed because it contains 6 times more calcium than the milk, 8 times more Omega 3 than the salmon, 30 times more antioxidants than the blueberries, 3 times more iron than the spinach, 15 times more magnesium than broccoli and 25% more fibers than the flex seed. Additionally, their carbohydrates get transformed slower into sugar. That means they are ideal for people who exercise because chia generates energy steadily and for a long time. All these qualities and the fact that they are easy to prepare by just soaking them into a liquid (milk, juice, water), make them a good choice to use at any time.

I was mentioning in the other chapter about the amount of proteins one individual needs to eat in a day in order to gain muscles. For growing muscle mass, an athlete needs to eat twice in protein grams of the weight amount he has. If a person weights 50 kg, he needs to eat 100 grams of protein per day. To count the grams per day we could use the table below. 100 grams of meat is about the size of an average palm. One regular cup of milk has 250 ml. All these quantities you will be able to figure out easy and have an idea how much you should eat. The table will show the protein quantity that exists in every 100 grams of a produce.

Food Type (100 grams)	Protein quantity (grams)	Complete protein
fish	19	yes
beef	25	yes
beef liver	20	yes
chicken	20	yes
organs	17	yes
goose	18	yes
turkey	23	yes
duck	20	yes
pork	20	yes
pork liver	19	yes
rabbit	22	yes
lamb	18	yes
sheep	17	yes

headcheese (toba de porc)	22	Yes
ham	18	yes
hard salami	25	yes
1 full egg (50 gr.)	6.5	yes
1 egg white	5	yes
milk	3.3	yes
farmer's cheese	16	yes
kefir	4.5	yes
pressed cheese	28	yes
raw cacao	20	yes
bee pollen	1.2	yes
quinoa	4	yes
beans	23	no
peas	21	no
lentils	25	no
poppy seeds	19	no
peanuts	25	no
sun flower seeds	27	no
pumpkin seeds	35	no
pistachio	22	no
walnuts	19	no

almonds	24	No
oatmeal flakes	13	no
rice	9	no

Usually, the fatty meats lose some of their proteins. Look for meat with not so much fat in order to bring more protein in the body per 100 grams produce. On the other hand, also the dairy products lose some of their protein when the fat is separated, during the manufacturing process.

If we look in the table, the headcheese has quite a large amount of proteins. Meat contains protein as well as the gelatin that is around. During the manufacturing process, the organs and/or meat is boiled for long time till the liquid in the pot gets sticky. When the liquid gets cold, the fat raises on top forming a fat layer. That layer can easily be scraped off. The gelatin underneath and the meat remain with much less fat. This is a source of protein too, but it is still not so healthy because it is a smoked product and it contains animal fats that should not be consumed too often and not into a large quantity. Otherwise, the fats that we eat are not so dangerous as the simple carbohydrates.
Even if the ham or salami have a good amount of proteins at 100 grams product, they are still not healthy

to eat in large quantities and for a long period of time. Even if we may find ham with no nitrates and nitrites, it may have too much salt and it is smoked. Smoked products release toxins in the body and we need a lot of work to clean it up. Moreover, at least in United States, I found this type of meats with honey or sugar added. The most disgusting food ever. This is my opinion only. Many people enjoy these types of tastes. The idea of eating so many simple carbohydrates on regular bases, it does not help.

Another example of food with high amount of protein is the pressed cheese. Unfortunately, it contains a lot of fat, too. We have to search for food high in protein and less fat or with no sugar added. Here it comes the role of the nutritional supplements and the protein concentrate or amino acids, where the protein comes separate from fats.

1.2. Carbohydrates

Always we have to make sure we do not eat too many simple carbohydrates or those who act like them. We should look for carbs with low glycemic index in order to keep the insulin level under control. Time to time as once per week, we may give a boost and eat a high glycemic carb but this should not be a rule and should not be too often.

On another hand, even if we eat complex carbs all the time, there is another factor which influences a diet – the combinations we do. It is not advisable to combine complex carbs with the oleaginous fruits. For example, the rice, pasta or bread (whole wheat or whole cereals) are good to be eaten separate of the time we eat almonds, peanuts, walnuts or seeds because the complex carbs from the first group of food associated with the healthy fats from seeds and nuts, it is an amount of calories way too high for our system to receive at one time. Our body will not be able to digest everything well and these foods will form fat deposits. Another combination that is heavy for our system to digest is the meat associated with bread, pasta, rice but also with the nuts and seeds. Another heavy combination is the fruits associated with any other food. These are big mistakes that bring that puffy look for the body and later on some cute ornaments will show up to the skin called cellulite. Off course, if only we do these combinations once in a while, we are not at risk of having cellulite. But, when these combinations are the norm for us all day long, every day, it is a high risk of being full of cellulite. If we also add beverages with sugar, we have the full recipe for cellulite and an unhealthy life style.

When we drink too much alcohol, our body cannot digest as usual the carbs coming from food. Our system needs to take care of the alcohol first and let the food to wait. This way the food is not processed in time and it transforms into fat. The alcohol does not contain lots of carbs but it slows the breaking down process of the other carbs. If we drink a small quantity of alcohol, it benefits us. Especially when we compete, alcohol gives you vasodilatation and it has other beneficial facts. Wine is known as a very good drink for the blood vessels. A natural wine is full in nutrients that feed the blood. Red wine contains melatonin, a sleeping aid and other antioxidants. It also contains the strongest antioxidant called resveratrol. This one exists in much higher quantity than in certain red plants as carrots or beets. Usually, the resveratrol exists in purple fruits or vegetables but in a smaller quantity than we find it in the red wine. It contains flavonoids which helps decreasing the bad cholesterol. The sweet alcohol drinks or the cocktails are not so good because they usually contain sugar. Sugar is 100% simple carb.

Fruits are healthy carbohydrates who bring a lot of benefits. They digest quickly and do not stay long into the stomach. That is the reason we need to eat them on empty stomach and not after a meal. When we eat them after consuming other food, they will stay too long in our stomach on the top of the other food. They will rot inside there and will produce gas and implicitly a bloated tummy. When the fruits and vegetables are consumed properly and they do not cause any health issue, they are good for the fibers, the vitamins and minerals contribution to our system.

As vitamin sources, we find Vitamin C in strawberries, oranges, grapefruits, kiwi, parsley, etc. Vitamin B9 exists in green bean pods, spinach, lettuce, peas, lentils, citric fruits, cereals and others. Vitamin K exists in cabbage, cauliflower, broccoli, spinach, etc. Another important antioxidant – vitamin A, it is found in the red vegetables as carrots and tomatoes, in the greens as parsley leaves and spinach and in colored fruits as apricots, peaches, oranges or yellow melon. Even if tomatoes are considered fruits, I personally cannot eat them into a fruit salad or separate them of a meal with proteins. The habitude is the second nature. That means when somebody has been using the same eating habits for all her/his life, it is very difficult for him to change that.

1.3. Fats

There are good and bad fats. Firstly, let's talk about the good fats that help our body to get rid of the bad cholesterol and bring so many other benefits. Reading a label on a product, we have to search for those products which have higher amount of **polyunsaturated fats and**

monounsaturated fats. These are the good fats. We can find these fats mostly in fish, olive oil and other type of healthy oils, avocado, nuts, flax or other seeds. We may take these fats from nutritional supplements under the form of pills or liquid – Omega 3, 6, 9. There are still studies that come contradictory about the benefit of these healthy oils for the cardiovascular system and our heart. They are definitely healthy oils for our system, but we cannot know for sure if they really help our heart. They do not damage anything anyway if we use them in a specific proportion. Before the researchers will demonstrate the opposite, we do not have another option but use Omega oils.   Additionally, the unsaturated fats help us to lose fat!!! Omega 3, 6 and 9 are good for enhancing the brain capacity, help with concentration, depression, mood, attention, patience and others. There are **saturated fats** which are called bad fats. They may increase the bad cholesterol inside the body especially in adults but they may help if we eat them with moderation during the winter season. In the last time, there are specialists who affirm that the bad fats do not form the bad cholesterol. Only the high glycemic carbs can do that. If a healthy person who does exercise regularly, eat a food containing saturate fat at one meal per month or per two months, it does not do any bad. We need even saturate fat for a correct functioning of our system but used in a small amount only. An average child that is not obese, needs unsaturated and saturated fats as well for a good development. Saturated fat exists in the whole milk, cheese, any meat (more or less), etc. Saturated fat helps our brain and the nervous system. It protects us to adjust our body temperature during the winter season or when we enter into a cold environment. When a person does not have a thick layer of fat to cover his body with, he will be too sensitive to cold but he will not suffer into a hot environment. I personally need much more fat on me for tolerating the rooms ventilated with the conditioned air during the summer. One of the fats that has a lot of qualities is the duck lard. Even if it is a lard, surprisingly, it contains 75% monounsaturated fat, 13% saturated fat, 10% Omega 6 and 2% Omega 3. The duck lard has less saturated fat than butter. Duck fat is closer nutritionally to olive oil but the difference is that the duck fat has a higher smoking temperature that makes it good for cooking. Another group of fats is the **trans fats** which are the worst and they should be avoided. They come from the fried food, salami, processed bakery products or certain margarines. Hydrogenated oils are very bad for the body. They are often used to preserve food and cans. Smoked foods are also bad because they form toxins and our body has to work very hard to get rid of them. Fried food is bad for us from the start and especially during the losing weight diets. When we want to do a mistake, at least we should do a smart one. We should fry food using an oil which smokes at a higher temperature. Examples of oils that burn at a high temperature and are good for cooking are: palm oil (232 degrees Celsius/ 450 F), avocado oil (271 C/ 520 F), refined sunflower oil (227 C/ 440 F), almond oil (221 C/ 430 F), peanut oil (231 C/ 440 F), refined corn oil (232 C/ 450 F).

As a general rule, it is not recommended to warm unrefined oils and those oils which are cold pressed. Even if they bring good nutrition for the body because of their healthy fats they contain, once we put them on top of the stove, their polyunsaturated fats become toxic and their smoking point become low. It is recommended that the unrefined vegetable oils to be used properly for the cold dishes to be able to benefit fully of their qualities. The smoking point of the oils refers to that temperature when these oils start to decompose their glycerin (smoking as a result of frying) and to release free radicals which are so harmful for our human system. The smoking point marks the beginning of oil degradation when the nutritional values get lost.

1.4. Pros & Cons

The majority of the food and drinks have benefits when consumed with moderation. As long as we eat and drink for the purpose of living and not just for the pleasure of eating, we will have a good long life. But when the food becomes an addiction and we live for the purpose of eating, the food and drinks may destroy us. We need to have a limit for the food quantity we eat. Drinking **coffee** brings many benefits to our system but using it in a too large quantity per day and every day, it may damage our health. Half a cup (1/2 of 250 ml) per day or at most 1 cup per day should be enough to wake you up for few hours and keep you sharp. We may use it for 2 weeks every day but we should do a break with it for the other following 2 weeks at least. This way the body do not get use to the coffee and you will feel its caffeine effect the times you drink it. There should be something bad about coffee, it is only the caffeine it contains when this is used for a longer period of time. But, caffeine acts as a pain killer and it helps for certain illnesses. There is also coffee without caffeine. Drinking coffee time to time, it helps. Coffee grain by itself contains a lot of antioxidants which renew the cells and help the body fight against diseases. Researchers found much more antioxidants in coffee than in fruits and vegetables for 100 grams product and they say it even reduces the risk for certain types of cancer because of this high quantity of antioxidants it contains. On another hand, too much caffeine may affect our heart, it takes out the Calcium from the bones and dehydrates, it lowers or raises the blood pressure in different cases for different individuals. When drinking coffee, we should also drink a lot of water to prevent dehydration. Dehydration lower the blood pressure and raises the heart rate in the same time. If we feel dizzy or faint after drinking coffee, this could be the reason. For all these health symptoms we should address everything to the doctor and keep in touch with a health care professional.

The salt may be both, friend and enemy. For the losing fat perspective, salt does not help. Many foods already contain salt. The easiest example is the egg. Do an experiment and try eating products with no salt in composition and do not add salt on the food or when cooking. In about one month you will notice the taste that many foods already have salt inside them as the egg has. At that point, a combination of egg with tomatoes, would make you discover how much quantity of salt exist into an egg, because the simple tomato does not have salt at all in her composition. When we are used to eat food that is high in salt, we are not able to distinguish certain tastes in the natural foods. Salami and pastrami contain too much salt, plus adding salt on top of other foods we eat, change our tasting ability. I was amazed when I saw my colleague dipping the already fried chicken thigh in a bunch of salt.

Too much salt as well as too low salt in the system, may give healthy issues as the risk for heart attack, stroke and high blood pressure. A low sodium level may decrease the aldosterone in the blood, a hormone that have a big influence for the cardiovascular system. In order to know your sodium level, it is always good to do some blood work and keep in touch with the doctor, to know if you need to add some salt on the food or not.

The egg is an important source of proteins and vitamins. It may be both good and bad for us. If we eat only the white, it brings us only benefits but if we do not add a little bit of yolk together, the protein from the white may not be absorbed in the system. Specialists recommend that we should eat couple or few whites with one or two yolks added. Another fact that a doctor recommended is to always eat the egg white cooked. When the egg is raw, it contains an antivitamin which eats the other vitamins inside the body. Moreover, he said that the egg has to be hard boiled or hard cooked for the bad cholesterol inside the yolk to be diminished at a minimum or even disappear. The soft egg yolk has the bad cholesterol. Its consume has to be limited.

Aspartame is a substance which replaces the sugar and helps us with the losing weight process. Unfortunately, aspartame is found as being carcinogen. Better use little sugar than aspartame. This is the most common and known artificial sweetener. There are many others which are unhealthy and need to be avoided.

1.5. Acid and Base

The human body cannot live without proteins because of many reasons. They help our system to build antibodies, defending it against viruses and bacteria and they have an important role for our breathing system. They are important for building the muscle mass we need. But on another hand, if we eat too much protein per day for years, we will have a lot of acid accumulation in our system. That is why, a regular person who does not do sport, does not sweat enough, does not drink enough water and not eat vegetables enough, he will not get rid of this acid. Too much acid in the body may cause the different illnesses or may develop unwanted masses or tumors. Please eat a lot of alkaline food to compensate the food which develops the acid in the body. Drink a lot of water which is slightly alkaline or regular water which has a neutral PH. A lot of regular water would dilute the acid in the body and in the blood, too. Our blood has a neutral PH 7.0. Then, we need food and drink that have PH at least 7.0, 7.3 to 9. PH 1 and PH 14 are the extremes when 1 is way too acidic and 13, 14 are way too alkaline.

Unfortunately, the acid in the body comes a lot from the toxins and chemicals in the air we breathe or many other factors that more and more we cannot avoid in our surroundings. At least we should struggle to take alkalinity from the food we eat, as much as we are still able to do it, in the environment existing nowadays. The main cause of many illnesses as cancer and others, in the society we live, is too much acid accumulation in our system. In order to neutralize the acid, here is a natural combination which is effective for treating different illnesses or for just cleaning our body. We may do it time to time for making sure our body does not become too acidic. In case of an illness, there are specific treatments using these 2 components: lemon and sodium bicarbonate or just sodium bicarbonate. Lemon is acid but when it gets into our stomach, it becomes base. The same it happens with all the citric fruits when we eat them on empty stomach. This is one of the multiple reasons that they are very healthy to eat them. For certain people who have acid reflux issues, the citric fruits cause problems before they arrive in the stomach. They do not have the chance to be transformed in base before causing problems in the esophagus. To avoid this issue, those people may do a trick and transform the lemon into base before it enters inside the mouth. If we mix the lemon with sodium bicarbonate into a glass, we will have a base composition ahead of time. We may add some water to fill up the glass and dilute the mixture. This way we do not have the strong bad taste of the sodium bicarbonate and should not create problems for the esophagus. If the glass is drunk all the way in short time and we move and walk around, the acid in the stomach will come out as a strong burb. Moreover, the sodium bicarbonate will clean the blood further in the system. The lemon will bring its healthy nutrients and vitamins so necessary for us.

An alternative for eating fruits and vegetables without to be harsh for the stomach is to boil or bake them.

Coffee produces acid in the stomach. We need to drink plenty of water around it to ensure the release of that acid. But, coffee helps with digestion in the same time, it helps us using the bathroom and cleaning the colon, fact that is very important for a good functioning of the body. Coffee is also a diuretic. For a person with no water retention, it dehydrates and he need to drink a lot of water along with drinking the coffee.

Butter is a food that is not considered good when fried because its smoking temperature is pretty low, but when consumed moderately as a spread and not fried, it has lots and lots of benefits. Butter is alkaline! The word "butter" comes from the butyric acid it contains. This is a fatty acid which is produced by the bacteria inside the intestines at the contact with fibers. When we do not eat enough fibers, it would be good the butyric acid to still exist inside. Butter helps with that. Moreover, there are studies on rats which show that the butyric acid prevents gaining adipose layer and increase the fat burnings. Additionally, butter contains conjugated linoleic acid (CLA) which helps with losing the adipose layer and it has also other benefits. Of course, not to forget about the saturated fat in the butter. This is the reason we have to consume it with moderation. Overall, the nutritional qualities exceed the defects. Researchers found that fats in butter protect the joints and strengthen the arteries that get weakened because the lack of sleep. The butter also contains vitamins and minerals. The butter is also good for the brain because of the oleic acid it contains. This fatty acid protects the neurons. Specialists say the butter contains also the good cholesterol. Moreover, it has some fatty acids which protect the stomach against the gastro-intestinal infections. All the milk products are alkaline and they offer so many benefits, especially those which contain more fat. Unfortunately, they lose many of their qualities with the pasteurization and homogenization procedures.

The important bacteria that benefit the body are the probiotics. We may find these good bacteria in kefir, in some types of yogurts or in homemade pickles or sauerkraut. On the other hand, there exist also prebiotics, which nourish the probiotics. The prebiotics are usually fibers which act like food for the good bacteria. Their existence makes the digestion much easier and decreases the inflammation in the colon. The prebiotics are transformed in the intestines in the fatty acid called butyric, an acid that also exists in butter, as mentioned earlier. It is helpful taking probiotics and prebiotics from pills as nutritional supplements, but our body can take them from the natural food as follows:
-prebiotics are in: asparagus, beans, peas, oatmeal, bananas, berries, dandelion, garlic, onion, leek.
-probiotics are in: sauerkraut or homemade pickled cabbage together with the liquid it stays in (moare de varza), homemade pickled green tomatoes (cucumbers, cauliflower, etc.), homemade yogurts or couple of store yogurts, kefir.

To take advantage of the benefits of probiotics, the fermented food and liquids must not be pasteurized. During the pasteurization process, those good bacteria get destroyed.

Usually, alkaline foods are the cooked vegetables,

vegetable juices, cooked and not cooked fruits, some cereals and dairy products. On the other hand, by cooking the veggies and the fruits, they lose some of the vitamins they contain. Moreover, if we add sugar in the water we boil the fruits, they become acidic. Dried fruits tend to be more acidic because they have a high concentration of sugar. The fruity sweet yogurts are acidic, as well. Uncooked citric fruits are acidic but once entering in the stomach, they become alkaline when they make us burb and release the gas out from the stomach. They are good for people without acid reflux issues, only. Alkaline inside our body also comes from happiness, calm, relaxation, physical and mental exercise, breathing exercises, good mood, joy, good deeds and day light. Acidic foods for the human body are the fried foods and meats, sweets, cakes, chocolate, artificial honey made from sugar, artificial fructose (not extracted from fruits), lactose, eggs, fish eggs, smoked food, vinegar, additives, colorants, alcohol, cocoa, pickles made with vinegar, mayonnaise, cigarette smoking, certain parfums and air fresheners, bleach spray, etc. Acidic environments are stress, not enough sleeping, sadness, hatred, anger and some medicines. Certain breads, bakery products and sugar are acidic, too. Some breads contain sugar transforming them into cakes. Bread is not good for us because the gluten and starch it contains. Eating doughs and breads make us want to eat more to the next meal.

The starch is converted too fast into sugar and it raises the glycemia (blood sugar). The gluten has similar feature as the glue. The gluten is not good for many people, not only for those who were diagnosed with celiac disease. We can find out if we are sensitive to gluten if we do not eat bakery products, bread or products with gluten for 2 weeks to 1 month and then try to eat bread. If after one month, when we start eating bread again, we will feel bloated, pain to the stomach, tired more than usual, digestive problems and/or other bad symptoms, it means we have gluten sensitivity and it is advisable to avoid eating bakery products as much as possible. Moreover, some of the whole wheat breads are not made from the real whole wheat. We are kind of screwed. Our ancestors were eating simple boiled pearl barley or raw wheat germs. They were much stronger and much healthier than we are today with our advanced manufactured and polished bread and other "high quality" products.

In the human body exist 2 liquids: blood and lymph. The blood transports the nutrients to the cells and the lymph transports the toxins to the certain organs for the purpose of being released out of the body. The lymph brings the toxins to the liver, kidneys and skin to push them out of the body. The largest organ, the skin, will be able to clean up everything with a little help. Unlike the blood, nobody pumps the lymph to move. We must push it or shake it to flow. This is the main reason we really need to exercise! If we do not exercise, the toxins remain in the body and they form an acidic blood. Our blood is base by nature. When it becomes acidic, it has time just about 4 minutes to turn back into base, otherwise the life of that body would stop. The blood must hurry up and neutralize its PH. In this emergency situation, he uses bases from the bones and teeth, the calcium and magnesium. But what does the body when he is not able to clean the blood up in few minutes? He throws all the acid on the cells. What does it happen if he throws with acid few times per day? Those cells may have two options. They may die or they may learn to live into an acidic environment with no oxygen. These are the cancer cells. Each of us have some of these cells more or less. Our immune system (the white cells) destroys them. But, the cancer cells are slick like any other enemy. They know to hide behind some healthy cells and the white cells are not able to see them. There are studies about the fact that usually, the cancer cells need many years or long time to multiply. That is why we need to figure out how we can have a long healthy life style. If during those many years we try fasting few times with no animal food or liquid, the white cells will be able to see again the bad cancer cells and they will destroy them. During a religious fast, God may heal us of cancer and we do not even know we had it! More and more people discover that chemotherapy kills both cancer cells but also healthy cells. Chemotherapy paralyzes the white cells, as well and we cannot rely anymore on our immune system. Good luck to a slightly alkaline lifespan!

Chapter 2

Muscle Mass

We are all different. Every one of us may have a different metabolism. Each body is able to assimilate the nutrients in its own way. Some of us could eat a lot of carbohydrates and the adipose layer does not increase. For others, the quantity of the carbohydrates must be limited because the thickness of the fat layer on top of their body gets increased much faster.

It is unbelievable for people who get fat quickly that, there are separate individuals who really wish to become big and grow in volume. Yes, there are. Their body system is called ectomorph. These are people who have a very fast metabolism. For them it is harder to gain weight.

There exist people with a combined body type as well. They have features belonging to both, endomorph and ectomorph types. For them gaining weight or losing weight is sometimes hard and sometimes easy. Of course, that may be influenced not only by their eating habits but, by the stress or the activities they are involved in, for days or for longer periods in life.

When we bring the idea of gaining weight into a discussion, everybody thinks first about the fact of becoming big, bulky does not matter what or how. It is very important to consider that gaining weight without having everything under control, can be unhealthy and it may bring cholesterol, blood pressure problems or many other health issues. Trying to gain weight by eating everything with no measure or pushing by force in our body a large quantity of food, it may even bring that body from an ectomorph type to an endomorph body type over few years of doing so. It will change his metabolism. It will enlarge one's stomach too much by forcing to push in it a large quantity of food at one time. His intestines will become large and the person's waist thick. That is because the body has to adapt with processing a large amount of food. Then, the same individual who earlier, was tormenting himself to eat a lot, he is starting now to torture his body to starvation after couple of years of eating a lot.

When gaining weight, the ideal is to gain muscles and not fat. Now, of course, the minimum level of fat for a human body to be healthy, is needed to exist at all time. When I personally speak about gaining weight or losing weight, I am not talking about the amount of the calories used. A human body needs calories in order to increase his own muscular mass and in order to lose adipose tissue as well. That means, we cannot speak in terms of calories when trying to have a diet.

A diet which fits to your personal needs is important when you have a goal, for both purposes of gaining weight or losing weight. When I mention the word diet, I am not referring to a strict one that an individual has to keep it for a while. I am referring to a way of life that creates your life style.

For gaining muscular mass, we need to use healthy food as well. "Big people" should be healthy, too. As I have learned, a lot of bulky people who have succeeded in gaining muscles, they have also accumulated a lot of fat with it. This is because all that they think is to grow, it doesn't matter what. Which is the purpose of having big muscles when nobody is able to see them because they are covered by a thick layer of fat. At that point, in order to discover your muscles, you need to start getting rid of the adipose layer on top. This process involves losing some muscles, too. When you lose fat, you lose some muscles with it. When you gain muscles, you could gain easy fat with it. Sometimes today but mostly in the past, athletes have believed that during the bodybuilding off season, in order to gain weight, it is good to gain also fat with it, to have the muscles covered underneath because they develop better this way. In my opinion this is a bad idea. Why should someone look good only couple of times per year at the competition times? Why couldn't we look good all the time? Gaining fat along with gaining muscles, destroys our health and the skin quality. Everybody gets older over time. If we increase the body volume and then decrease it many times, after years of keep modifying our mass, the skin will be additionally affected. The skin loses its natural elasticity with the age. We do not want to add more damage to it. Additionally, where is a big volume of anything, muscles or fat, all the organs in the system including the heart have to work more than the normal pace. That would force them to struggle sometimes for no reason.

This book is meant to serve for a regular individual, too. It is not only for competitors. That is why I need to mention the last comment is referring to a regular person as well, who has weight issues when he gains or loses weight many times in a life span. It does not matter what type of weight there is, fat or muscle. When it is too much mass, the skin stretches around and the time when that mass disappears, it seems we have too much skin hanging.

We all need muscles for regular activities in our life or to be able to move. But we also need muscles for helping us to lose the unwanted fat. It is said: as much muscles you have, as easier you will be able to get rid of the fat. On another hand, too much muscles could work against. They could make us become quite rigid, not flexible and big muscles are at risk of becoming petrified with aging. Than the big guy is starting to have muscular cramps more often and the massage sessions are expensive, plus your partner does not have time to give a massage every moment you are in need. Although, the massage helps indeed in those type of situations. In a competition, a big ripped muscular mass is spectacular but every enjoyment in life have both regrets and pleasure.

Any sport if done in a professional way involves risks but also benefits. At a competitional level, each sport can be dangerous and not healthy. But, if you went through and you escaped in good conditions being able to recover, it is worth it. You look back with confidence, concluding that your struggle gave yourself mental balance, strength to go forward and a tone of information that no one can steel from you. Only the time and the fact you would not share that information with anyone else, it could make you lose that luggage full of knowledge.

When someone is ectomorph, it is difficult for him to gain muscular mass but he cannot be afraid about gaining fat. That is why, he is allowed to eat more food. He may do eating mistakes more often. He will burn and consume the sugar faster. This does not mean he should eat all kind of unhealthy foods at all time. His cholesterol might increase too, even if his body looks thin. He might develop other illnesses as the time passes. Moreover, the energy which comes from simple carbohydrates or bad food does not have the same quality as the one which comes from the complex carbs. When you exercise and do not eat healthy, your workout will not be so lucrative. As you start eating qualitative food (see Chapter 1 about qualitative food meaning), you will see an increase in your workout quality, followed by the enhancement in muscle quality.

As an ectomorph type human body, you should eat more proteins, carbs and even fats. Please see examples of programs for gaining muscular mass in the Chapter 4 of this book. Along with the examples, that chapter will describe how, why and when we are allowed to do mistakes in our eating habits.

For an ectomorph individual, it is also advisable to consume mostly complex carbs but, they should be ingested in larger quantities than an endomorph. It is important the break time of 2 hours between meals. This interval should be respected in order to leave enough time for the system to assimilate the food. Even if an ectomorph may digest faster the nutrients, his system still needs time for food procession.

Earlier I was mentioning the fact of not counting the calories in our diet. We should rely on counting proteins and carbs in our eating habits when we wish to build muscles. For example, a slice of chicken breast contains 20 grams of proteins. Then, an ectomorph person could eat 2 slices (40 grams) of chicken breast per meal as source of protein. Concerning an endomorph type who digests slower and may gain adipose tissue much easier, he may eat only 20 grams of meat per meal. This is because the meat has in composition not only protein. The fat from the meat may not be so useful for the person who gains weight easy. Even if carbohydrates are more dangerous than fats in the gaining fat issue, we also need to be careful about the amount of fat we eat. If an endomorph individual eats 2 slices of meat per meal, theoretical he builds muscles with one slice and the other slice is deposited somewhere as an unwanted layer on his body. In order to gain muscles but not fat in the same time, you have to eat small amount of food but many times per day with 2 hours brake in between like babies do. It is imperative that the total amount of protein per day consists in regular food along with nutritional supplements: protein powder or simple amino acids. By supplementing the protein intake in a day, we are able to keep under control the fat and carbs quantity as well.

In order to build muscle mass, a person needs to eat twice the amount of protein grams as his bodyweight is. That means, when a person's weight is 100 kilograms in total, he must eat at least 200 grams of proteins. See the table for the amount of proteins contained in 100 grams of food product. If a person does not exercise, most likely he will gain fat with no muscles when eating this much. Muscles do not form by themselves or by laying in bad and watching TV. Nor by transforming fat into muscles as some of the people would believe. Muscle mass grows by eating healthy food, resting and exercise. A lucrative workout cannot last only 5 or 10 minutes as some people do. The workout with weights has to take between 30 minutes and 45 minutes/ session. If you exercise more than 45 minutes, the muscles will be over worked and in other words, you will start to kill them. In that case, your body will not answer the way you want, because you stress it too much. Keep in mind that what is too much, it is indeed too much. If you beat a hen to lay more eggs, she will get mad and she won't lay at all in the best case. But the worst it is when she might die. We do not want to kill the hen!!!

After 30 minutes of lifting weights, the testosterone level is increased at the maximum. After 45 minutes, it starts to decrease. Over 60 minutes the testosterone comes back to its initial level.

Even if we want to grow muscles, it would be recommended to continue doing cardio exercise, bicycle, running, swimming, etc. Indeed, running every day or twice per day when we want to gain muscles, it is not indicated. But, running one or two times per week it is beneficial. By doing some cardio too, the blood flow gets increased. That will help the system to do its job easier, the nutrients to reach the cells who are in need and then the muscles will be excited to grow. During running you see the mass volume increasing. But do not let yourself fooled by that. That only means, the muscles are pumping more blood for the moment and they will get back to the initial volume as before. The same it happens when you exercise with weights. The muscles look bigger for the moment. Building qualitative muscles is a long process which involves good eating habits, nights with sleep and discipline.

Another factor which helps and it is mandatory for building muscular mass is taking nutritional supplements. In the NS Chapter, I will explain thoroughly about the time when these nutritional supplements must be taken and the reason. I will explain as well the types that are

needed to be taken before, after the workout or during different moments in the day or night. If in need of building muscles, it is useful to take powder protein with a percentage of 50% protein at 100 grams product.
As an ectomorph person type, it is not bad to use time to time a product with more carbs especially taken after workout. Let's say a product containing 70% carbs and 30% proteins. But, do not forget the proteins are the building blocks for gaining muscles. That means, it is imperative to use the proportion of 2/1 (2 grams of protein/1 kilo body mass).

If we are very active throughout the day, we also need a good amount of carbohydrates. This is because carbs serve as the main fuel for energy. If we do not eat enough carbs, our system will take its energy from proteins or fats. We need proteins for building muscles and not for using them as source of energy. Moreover, when taking energy from proteins, our body will struggle having more work to do. The system will need to transform the proteins in glucose first and then in energy. This is a longer process than in the carbs case. That means we have to wait little longer before feeling energized.
If we do not eat enough but we exercise a lot, our muscles will enter in catabolism mood. They will not grow, nor stay the same. In this case, the muscles will get smaller, they will atrophy.

The ketogenic diets for losing fat, when eating zero carbs or too little bit of carbs, it brings loss of muscle mass. In this case it is recommended for one day per week to eat carbohydrates to replenish the glycogen reserves. Some body builders use this method in their despair of not having enough time to lose all the necessary fat before competition. But, this diet brings them with less muscle mass on the stage. On another hand, when using unnatural products, the process changes. The amino acids are quickly taken straight to the muscles and they do not enter in the catabolic state.

Another factor which could stay against the muscles growth is stress. Stress develops some catabolic hormones. When we are stressed out, our system uses some of the proteins we are eating, to repair the damage which is caused by the catabolic hormones. Then, some proteins go towards recovery, instead of being used as building blocks to gain muscles. The same it happens when we are sick. Our body uses the nutrients for health recovery, being harder for the muscles to grow. Stay healthy! This is the main condition of building muscles.

It is mandatory for building muscles to work out with big weights. But it is more important to do the exercise correctly. Here it is little tricky because surprisingly, many of us do not know how to execute correct all the exercises. Unfortunately, I have seen trainers who do not show to their client the correct way of doing the exercise. In US nowadays, a regular person needs some luck to find a knowledgeable trainer. My advice would be to look for trainers who have entered in competitions and have already received more than one medal. This in case the first one was won by having no other competitors present with him on the stage. It is sad when the strong point of a trainer is to count the seconds of those 2 minutes break between the sets for his client or to change the pin on the weight lifting machine.

Be lucky and find a good trainer who have the experience and the knowledge that you can trust. If you want to compete in the future, it would be good to form your own luggage of knowledge fit with your body, picking up advice from different sources. Learn how your body respond to different changes that you are attempting to do.

If you do not work out correct, some of your fibers could be left aside. Then, they will not be developed at their full capacity. More over working out incorrectly could bring accidents and irreversible problems to the spine. In the chapter "Exercise types" I will try to explain as good as I can in writing, the correct way of doing the exercises. It is easier to understand when somebody is showing to you face to face, but you will surely have an idea of a correct execution for the basic exercises.

The heavy and correct lifting is important but there are times when we do have different muscular or joint problems. Those times we can maintain our muscular mass and definition by posing a lot. If you exercise your muscles to stay often in a certain position, they will learn to be in that shape. On another hand, we should keep track of our posture. Please notice if your shoulders tend to stay hunch or the upper body have the tendency to lean in a side too often. These may become severe problems over the years and we may grow muscles on a bad and unhealthy skeleton. If your toes are directed inwards when you are a child or a young man and you do not correct that soon, the knees will go inwards and the hips will be modified. The same thing happens when we keep the toes too outwards. An incorrect posture will affect the spine and our muscle structure will form on that frame. Even if we gain muscle mass, at that point, we are looking bad and not healthy. I was observing some individuals like this, with a bad posture. Even if they have built muscle mass and they are working out hard, they are not so handsome in front of the ladies because of their posture.

A way of growing muscle mass is to shock the body system by alternating 2 weeks of less carbs in your diet with other 2 weeks when the amount of carbs is high. A competitor is growing his muscle mass after each competition. Before the competition, he follows a strict diet low in carbohydrates and after competition, his body explodes in gaining muscles by introducing in his off season diet more carbs. Two weeks period is not too long for those carbs to be transformed in fat deposits. When the body realizes there are too many carbs for the system and he will decide to do deposits of adipose layer, we will shock it right in time by reducing drastically the amount of carbs. This way the system will not make deposits of fat. On the other side, when we eat mostly protein and not much carbs or not even any for 2 weeks, the body system will not have time to realize what is going on and he will not enter in catabolism before 2 weeks. The muscles will be depleted of carbs and when reversing the diet, the muscles will be hungrier for glycogen and they will absorb the upcoming carbs. Those carbohydrates form the necessary energy and they will not go as fat deposits.

During the off season, having a thick adipose layer does not help because the level of myostatin gets increased. That brings a low anabolic effect or even a not existent one. When we lose fat, the myostatin decreases, too. Than it is easy to gain muscle mass. It is advisable, when we are at diet, we should try doing almost the same heavy lifting, at the same intensity as the times we are not at diet, to help maintaining and growing the muscular mass. All these mentioned, they reflect the fact that there are certain times when our body is more able to grow its muscle mass. That period is after a diet, for example, after a competition the anabolic effect is huge because we start eating more carbs when the muscles are hungry. I personally believe, we do not have to keep this loading period longer than 2 or 3 weeks because the myostatin level will start to increase. During a diet, our fat level is low. That means the myostatin level is low. After the diet, the myostatin does not increase its level right away. It needs a while to wake up. Before it wakes up, we have to work out at gaining the muscle mass.

Another factor which may influence in a way to increase your amount of muscles is stretching. This helps the body not only to maintain a good flexibility but also to break out short pieces of your fibers. When these fibers recover, they become thicker and they add and develop new ones around them as a defense mechanism. The muscles are guided by the fundamental truth - what does not kill you, it makes you stronger.

The same way it happens when we exercise with heavy weights. The difference is that the muscles are forced much more, then the recovery will build more muscle tissue. Some of the fibers are breaking. When they recover, they become stronger and develop new ramifications.

The workout for gaining muscle mass consists in lifting heavy weights with less repetitions per set. You should pick up the weights which are as heavy as you can do 6 to 8 repetitions during 4 sets apart. Two minutes long should be the resting break between the sets. If you rest more than that because your workout colleague is talking too much, do not listen to him. When those two minutes ended, start a new set. If you take a too long break between the sets, your muscles get cold because the blood flow gets slower in the part of the body you work on. Then it comes the risk for accidents, overstretching or even muscle and tendon breakage. Then you will not be able to work out for weeks or months. The number of the sets for gaining muscular mass is usually 12 for each large group of muscles and 9 for each small group of muscles. It means you can do 4 types of exercise with 3 sets each or 3 types of exercise with 4 sets each for a big group of muscles. For a small group of muscles, you need to do 3 types of exercises with 3 sets each or 2 types of exercises with 4 sets each.

Now, in case we start to get sick, for example to catch a cold, we could lower the number of sets and just exercise to feel comfortable, without straining. Usually, when we see the first signs of a cold, we could go to the gym. The body and mind might recover because we raise the blood flow by exercising. But if the cold has already gotten too far in its cycle, we feel weak and feverish, it is not a good idea to go to the gym because whichever energy we still have at that point, we need to conserve it. The body will use it for the healing process. The nutrients in your body would go where it is needed for healing first anyway. For that moment, they will not go to the muscles. The first condition for growing our muscular mass is to be healthy and make sure we stay healthy at all time.

Every person is different but each of us have a certain amount of red fibers and an amount of white fibers. God left everybody on Earth with different abilities which serve for separate purposes. Some of us are built with more red fibers which are longer and thinner and are made for having running resistance and stamina. Those people are certainly made for running and sports where cardio is mainly used. They develop harder a big muscular mass. There are people with more white fibers. Those people have muscles which get developed easier in volume, in mass. These people are good for bodybuilding and power lifting. Their muscles are shaped shorter and thicker. The ideal for a complex bodybuilding development is when the individual has both type of fibers, in proportion of approximately 70% white fibers and the rest red fibers.

It is a good habit to use complex carbohydrates all the time. Even if you look for increasing your muscle mass, it is not a good idea to eat mostly simple carbs or carbs that have very high glycemic index as sugar. They give too much energy right away but soon all this energy will be gone. Complex carbs or those carbohydrates who act like them, give energy for a longer period of time. We should love these types of carbs because they make us feeling energized for a while. They allow you to consume the amount of energy little by little. We have to avoid as much as possible the simple carbohydrates with high glycemic index because they increase at first the insulin level in our body too quick and they decrease the insulin even less than initially, afterwards. In nowadays society, when we are already confident we have money saved up to be enough for our kids' college and for retirement, the financial crisis is coming and all of a sudden, not only that we lose all the money we have saved in investments but the inheritance from our parents as well. Better have less but permanent income than none. The same way, it works with our insulin, too. We do not have to raise the insulin too high because it will drop even lower than before. Depressing but true. Love complex carbs!... or better said food with low glycemic index.

For gaining muscular mass we should raise our natural testosterone. There are many tips that help raising the natural testosterone. Having a diet low in carbs for 3 weeks for example, followed by a week of more carbs included, it helps with a boost of testosterone. If you have already competed, you know that after the severe diet for the contest, you gain much easier and good quality muscle mass. Mainly, we should workout the basic exercises in order to increase the natural testosterone level. All the fancy exercises that many people have started to do in the gym for the last few years, do not help. Those are probably good for stretching only and for some blood flow. It is definitely better than stretching in bed! But, in order to grow the muscle mass, we have to work out much more seriously doing the basic types of exercise with free weights as squats, deadlifts for hamstrings and glutes, deadlifts for all the body (these are the regular deadlifts), rows with a bar for the back, bench press for chest, bench press with a bar for triceps and others. See the "Exercise Types" chapter for all the main exercises and their description. Theoretically, we have to increase our strength and lift little heavier week after week. This way our muscles have a thriving development. Not all the time it happens as we plan. Like any other thing, we may have good times and bad ones. Sometimes we get sick or we are stressed out because of our life encounters. Many time, we need to take it almost from the beginning but our strong will, gives us strength to start all over. We need a lot of years of perseverance to build muscle mass.

The last couple of reps within a set are the most important ones. Do not be lazy to do them. Those are the hardest but they have a crucial impact for your muscle growth. The last rep should be the one that after it, you cannot do any other rep. Only this way you can grow! Leave the machines for when you have a bad day and you are not in the mood for having a serious workout.

Everything what you eat after workout is going to build muscles. Right after the workout take a nutritional supplement or even two for a quick absorption. After half an hour we should eat regular food. We need to take advantage of this hour right after our workout when the system absorbs the most nutrients for building muscles. We do not have to exaggerate by eating a too large quantity of food though. The stomach needs to be able to digest everything within the 2 hours that follow the workout. Otherwise we might gain some fat, too. If we have a too full stomach, our body will need few hours to be able to break down all the food elements. In order to grow, we need amino acids which are the building blocks and carbohydrates to replenish the glycogen lost during the heavy lifting workout. If you decide to take two types of nutritional supplements after your workout, an example would be: 5 mg (1 teaspoon) of glutamine right after your workout. Leave a pause of 10 or 15 minutes for that glutamine to absorb separately and then take another supplement if you wish. After those 10 minutes, you may take a whey protein shake with 50% to 75%

carbohydrate. After another 15 to 20 minutes you may start eating your regular food with both proteins and carbs. It is said that right after workout (about 25 minutes) is not good to eat regular food because the liver is still busy with the glycogen production. It is advisable to take some nutritional supplement(s) first, which are already broken down. This does not give so much work for the liver. It is easier for the stomach and liver to process it. It is advisable to take amino acids or protein concentrate after workout and not before. The liver uses the elements he receives in order to firstly produce energy for the body as a whole. This is the reason we must not avoid eating carbohydrates. Only the rest will be directed towards the muscle development. If we consume protein before exercise, the liver transforms it in glucose for hepatic glycogen as energy instead of using it for gaining muscles. It would be good to take protein supplements after workout and/or few or at least couple of hours before exercise. This way that protein will not be waisted and it will be directed to the specific muscles we have just worked out.

Some people separate the muscle groups within a day, working out two times per day. For example, in the morning working chest by itself and in the evening doing biceps. This is not a bad idea if you have time to do so. This way you could gain two high absorption periods within one day. Your groups of muscles will develop separately. This should not be bad, especially if you want to compete at a high level. It is not advisable to work out in the evening right before going to bed. Your adrenaline released during the workout and the high blood flow will not allow you to have a good sleep. It is recommended to workout not later than 7.30 pm when you go to bed at 10 pm. Allow your body to enter in the resting mood!

It is unavoidable to use heavy weights when working out in order to grow your muscle mass. But, it is also important to exercise correctly. Do not swing for doing your reps with a too heavy weight for you. This way you are forcing your joints unreasonably and accidents could happen much easier, plus the exercise will not be so efficient to fulfill your purpose. The results will not be so thriving for long term. Proceeding with a bad form for your reps, you do not focus anymore on one group of muscles. Many other muscles are involved this way and we cannot develop a nice shape. It is true, we need to force once in a while and swing our body little bit to workout with the heaviest weight for us, but this would be an exception which must not be used on a regular basis. Usually we have to stay within a correct technique. When I see people in the gym forcing themselves to work incorrectly their reps with too heavy weight for them and raising the risk for back damage, my skin gets goose bumps. I am very worried that over a short or a longer period of time that person would suffer of bad spine pain and he will still not look as good as he wishes.

Working out the main big muscle groups of the body, we will maintain and develop the other muscle groups. Especially when you do not have time so many days per week for going to the gym, you should focus on the main groups: chest, back and legs. By working our legs, we are maintaining other muscle groups as well. Legs are a big group of muscles. When we are working them, we stimulate an invasive blood flow which helps the whole muscular system existing on the body frame.

Try working out different groups of muscles during two consecutive days or within the same day. For example, during the same workout you should not combine chest with triceps. After training chest, you will not have enough strength for training the triceps. The chest exercise involves the triceps usage as well. It is advisable to work chest with biceps and back with triceps. Moreover, you may choose to train the legs on the day between the chest with biceps day and the back with triceps day. Additionally, you could train legs on the day between the chest, back days and arms, shoulders days. Usually, you have to leave a day off between 2 training days.We have to choose good combination for giving to each group of muscles the strength to be able to be worked out at its full capacity and leave enough time to recover and grow. If we work out the same group of muscles every day or during two consecutive days, we will not give it the chance to recover and develop properly. The muscles grow at home and not at the gym! After a heavier workout or a change in your exercise or when exercising after a break, you may have muscular fever. I am personally happy when I feel muscle fever. But, for some of us this is bothering. When the fever is too severe, you could do the same type of workout in the following day. That should help. Doing a hot bath is another method to get rid of the muscle fever.

It is very important to keep track of our age. An older person's body does not respond the same as the one of a young man. Even if the individual has been exercising all his life and his muscles are developed and he is used to a healthy life style, after a certain age, his body does not act the same. Then we have to do the necessary changes and not force our body on a too severe diet and not to eat big quantities of food to gain muscle mass. Those times we have to maintain what we have, only. Especially after 45 or 50 years old, the testosterone level decreases for a regular man, the joints and bones may become more fragile. Also, we are not so fast and quick in movements anymore. We may believe in our mind we are fast, but the reality is different. An older person may think he is lifting his legs during running at the same pace and height as before but, he may be surprised when he trips and falls this time without knowing why this is happening. Everybody goes through the same process: birth, growth and old age. Each time period has its advantages and disadvantages and we have to adjust because of them.

Chapter 3

Weight loss

Nowadays everybody has free access to power. We should be able to keep our weight under control by ourselves all the time. We should read more and start to think. Information gives you power. Try to take information from different sources, different nutritionists, dieticians, healthcare professionals and take advantage of the multiple sources on the internet or ask personal trainers. But, the most important is to start thinking. You must find tips and healthy diets which fit to your own body. No one else is able to know your body system better than you and find the right niche for you to lose weight. During the first month any diet functions.

But after a month or two, it is possible that your body may not answer to the same diet you have started. That is a sign you have to change something in your diet or in the way you exercise. After you pass that step, it will come another hard moment when you would like to be even more defined, in order to see yourself with pack abs and having more or less fibers on the body, when you see yourself in the mirror. As a female, you may decide how much of those fibers you like to uncover from underneath and when you would like to do so. But first you need to give yourself that choice. As a male, of course I wish you are able to form and uncover lots of fibers with a huge muscle mass in the same time.
It was believed that the muscles develop better under the fat. My opinion is we should look good all the time and do not put the body in a strenuous process of losing a lot of fat in a short period of time, when we could work at maintaining a thin layer of necessary fat and still see some lines and curves on your body permanently. Also, it is possible to gain muscles and in the same time to lose fat.

Firstly, we may start the losing fat process by reducing the amount of food we ingest. When we eat a lot, the stomach organ is enlarged, as well as the intestines. In order to have a thin waist we have to narrow the things that are inside of the body.

Start eating less per day. We must reduce the food quantity for each meal. The diet we eat has to contain all kinds of different foods but less amount of them. When we finish each meal, we have to still feel hungry a little bit. Feeling full at your stomach at the end of the meal is a mistake. In 10 minutes after you left the table, you will have the feeling of saturation anyway. The food needs 10 minutes to settle in the stomach and get mixed with water and your stomach fluids. The digestion process starts from the mouth when the food is chewed and mixed with saliva. Even if this is a world with rush and stress, please take your time and chew your food good enough, not to choke but to also leave an easier work to do for your stomach. Then, the digestion process will be much quicker.

For losing fat, the individual must eat often. Eat at least 5 meals per day. We should eat a meal once per 3 hours. Our body must trust us and see he receives fuel. If he sees he does not receive food time to time regularly, he will get scared. The body might think... he will never receive food. That is why the body is starting to gather deposits to make sure he will have some for later, too. An employee who receives his salary with delay, he is afraid he might not have enough money for living until his next pay check. Then, he goes to the bank and open a savings account. The difference is the savings account is good forever but the layer of fat only for the winter time!

We can get rid of the soft blanket which covers our muscles by reducing the grams of carbohydrates we ingest. It is advisable to reduce it descending, not suddenly. In the first 2 weeks we start by reducing little bit the amount of carbs, followed by the week 3 and 4 when the carbs amount should be even less. We should never get rid of the whole amount of carbs in our diet as the carbohydrates are the main source of energy. After one month of diet, you should feel a difference but after 2 months of diet, you will see a body shape that you should be proud of. Because of the changes that you do in your eating habits for the first 3 weeks, you will feel weird. Your body and mind will feel different but you are ok. Keep doing what you do and your body will get used to the new life style. In short time you will feel much healthier and more energized.

For your system to have an easier digestion, you need to try eating the different types of food as separate as possible and stop eating before feeling full to your stomach. It is advisable to separate carbs apart of the proteins for few meals and whenever is convenient for you. The human body processes different the proteins than the carbs. As well as different type of proteins take longer time to be digested and others less time. In order to make it easier for the body, it would be good to separate the food categories with 2 hours apart. This is not a mandatory solution for losing fat but it helps. This is for an easier digestion. There are certain diets which are working on this principle. You can find different types of diets into one of the next chapters.

Another factor that occurs when eating different types of food together is bloating. In general, almost all body types can suffer because of this condition at one point more or less. Eating unorganized gives you gas and water retention. The bloating delays the digestion process. It will slow the losing fat process. Because of this, you may have a thick waist and big belly but the main reason is not the fat tissue.   A second factor which causes to become bloated is eating certain foods which some body systems does not digest correctly. One category of food which could make you bloated is dairy. Milk products give a lot of gas in the stomach for those who have lactose intolerance. More over milk products make the body to retain water between the muscles and the skin. Then the individual will have a puffy aspect. Of course, milk products are good for calcium or proteins they contain but we may find lactose free milk products as well.

Above I was mentioning about the carbohydrates reduction during the process of losing fat. There are competitors or even regular people who reduce to zero the amount of carbs in their diet in order to lose fat faster. This way their body uses the fat as source of energy. That process is called ketosis. Even if ketosis seems an ideal procedure, I personally do not agree with this method because it might not be very healthy by forcing our system to proceed little different than its natural way. In addition, even if the method promotes the idea that the energy would come from fat, surely the energy is also coming from proteins and this is a waste. Even when using this method, I would not recommend to be used for a long period of time.

It is known that **fat burns on the carb's flame**. The basic of the old school of building a nice and healthy body still remains in place.

It may take years of discipline which you have to impose yourself on your own. Over the years, the individual gets used to this discipline and it will not be hard anymore at that point to keep a diet. That will come natural and easy as a way of life. Then, the environment will not influence you anymore. If the work mate or a friend offers you some cookies, you will be able to refuse those with no worries. At that point, if you see in front of your eyes a lot of good food, you will not be able to eat it because once the food gets into your shrunk stomach, you will get sick, nauseous, you will want to throw up. This may happen only when your stomach got small. It may take years before you will be this way and a little bit of food will be enough to make you feel full in the stomach.

Doing changes in your life or in your diet needs an iron will. We can build this will! A person who cannot start or continue a diet is weak. One of the benefits of the religious fasting along with getting healthy, it is making the man's will strong. Time to time it is good to fast, even if that means to take out of your diet all the animal products (proteins and fats). Two weeks of avoiding the animal proteins (meat, milk, cheese, eggs) does not have a big impact in losing muscle mass. But, it gives you a lot of mental will and it cleans your body of free radicals. That is very important for your system in order to function perfect and answer to your demands as the losing fat.

Hungriness is a necessity. It tells that you are healthy and your body needs nutrition. But, craving is a mental issue. Hungriness is a true feeling, craving is a false feeling. Many times, we eat to feel the pleasure and not because we feel hungry in the stomach. Moreover, sometimes we may feel empty in the stomach even if we have just eaten half an hour earlier. That it is another false sensation. That happens because we have forgotten to drink water.

The water is another important factor in our diet. Our body is made by 80% water. If we do not give enough water to our system, it will dry. We will dry inside and outside, including the skin. That is also a reason for the skin wrinkles.

The main condition for the losing fat process is too drink 2 liters of water per day for a 50 kg. bodyweight and 3 liters of water per day for a 100 kg. body weight. If we drink more than 4 liters of water per day, we will force our kidneys. When we are drinking a large quantity of water in the same time, again we force the kidneys. If we drink less than 2 liters of water per day, the level of toxins will increase in our body and the residues will not be flushed out. Water pushes the existing water out. We have to drink so much water until our urine is very light in color. If this is dark yellow, it means the urine is too concentrate in toxins. Of course, we have to consider, the urine color may be influenced by certain medicine we take or certain food. For example, we may have dark yellow urine when we take a lot of vitamins B (50 mg per each B vitamin) or red color when we eat beets. I personally do not feel I am thirsty most of the time, but if I do not force myself to drink enough water per day, I may start to feel sick and light headed. This is because I would become dehydrated without feeling thirty yet. When we are dehydrated, the blood pressure gets too low and the heart rate high. We may feel dizzy and the activity of the brain gets limited. We may not be able to focus when learning. We might wake up in the night with a very strong cramp on a certain muscle because of dehydration. After a little while of forcing our body to drink more water, our system gets used to this idea and it will ask for more water by itself. Sometimes when we feel thirsty, it is too late. It means the body is already dehydrated. That is the reason to drink water before having the feeling of thirst.

Our system accumulates free radicals from very many sources: not having a good diet, the fruits and vegetables can be full of pesticides and chemicals, pollution, stress, smoking, the heating/AC units in the house and others. Many things bring chemicals inside our body and are not good for our system. They form free radicals what we call toxins. If we cannot get rid of these toxins in time, our cells will get sick and it will be hard for our body to get rid of the fat, as well. We should not neglect the bad idea of fried food. It forms toxins in our body as well. That brings a good contribution to your cellulite. There are different ways to clean the system out of these toxins. As I have mentioned earlier, drinking a lot of water is the most important thing. But, when doing that, we really need to be careful because along with the toxins, we flush out of the body the vitamins and minerals. That may cause dizziness, muscle cramps and other side effects. Please start taking multivitamins and minerals daily when drinking a large quantity of water.
Another way to get rid of the toxins, it is sweating. During a diet it is recommendable to use sauna once or

twice per week but not mandatory. You can sweat by doing cardio exercises as running, jump rope, using the bike, swimming or different other sports, multiple times per week. It is advisable to do a combination of cardio types, to work the body from different angles.

A person who wants to lose fat should do more than walking. I saw many people just walking on treadmill or on the street. Yes, walking is good for blood circulation, but not for losing fat. By just simple walking you might lose little bit of weight but that is almost equal to zero. You will never reach the shape you like by only walking in natural conditions. It is advisable to walk for losing weight only when you are an obese individual for the purpose of not damaging your joints. A person with a big amount of fat or a huge muscular mass should walk only and do the weight lifting as a cardio. After 2 months, when that person lost a lot of weight and he feels comfortable doing more, it would be good for him to start other type of aerobic exercises. He might try running as well, if he has already lost enough weight at that point and he does not feel pain in the joints. **Running is the basic.** No other cardio exercise helps so much as running does. Moreover, running stays as a base for any sport. Does not matter what sport you do, if you include running in your training, you will see better results. Even if you practice chess only, running also helps you, by increasing the blood flow into your brain.

(I have meant this as a joke but it is actually a reality.)
If you are in the process of losing fat, you should run at least 4 times per week. It would be helpful to run every day or even 2 times per day. If you run so many times, it is mandatory to take vitamins. Along with the toxins, fat and some muscles, you will lose a lot of vitamins and minerals by running. Replace them with new ones. The vitamins that we take from food are not enough to replenish the ones lost. We should buy additional vitamins and minerals in the pill or liquid form.

When running, the duration of losing fat does not stop in the same time with the end of the running session. Your body continues to lose fat for another hour after you stop running.

It is more helpful to run 2 times per day for 20 minutes each, than 1 time per day for 40 minutes. Why having only 1 hour of losing fat, when we can have 2 hours of losing fat with the same amount of effort? Every running session has its separate process during our long weight loss period. At each time, during the first 10-15 minutes of running, we lose the glycogen from the muscles only. We start to lose fat after 10 to 15 minutes of running. That means, if we are running for 15 minutes only, we do not lose fat. The person is losing fat after the first 15 minutes and before 40 minutes of running. If we run more than 40 minutes in continue, we start to lose muscles. Our body will enter in catabolism.

We may run inside a gym on a treadmill or outside. I recommend running outside for the best results. Outside it is more oxygen. The fat gets burned in the presence of the oxygen only. There is more effective to exercise aerobically into an environment with more oxygen. The most effective time for doing cardio is in the morning on empty stomach or after the weight lifting workout. The muscles are already depleted of glycogen during those times and you are going to start losing fat from the beginning of your running. Doing cardio, you will lose some muscles anyway, as well. That is why it is recommended to take L-carnitine with 15 minutes before the running session and minimize the muscle loss. If we lose our muscles, it will be even harder for the system to lose fat.

When we are at the gym, if we start our workout with running followed by weight lifting, we will consume all the glycogen from the muscles. When it comes the time for weight lifting, we will not have enough strength and we will get exhausted sooner. That means, the fibers will not be worked out enough to be able to grow.
People may do a warm up on the treadmill for 5 minutes. That is fine. That helps the blood flow. But, this is different than a long running of half an hour which chases another purpose.

During a workout for losing weight, it is advisable to use easier weights and many repetitions. The weight should be as easy as you can do 12 to 18 repetitions in a set. The number of sets will be the same 4, as during the gaining mass program. The repetitions should be done much faster serving as a cardio session. The above idea of working out is not bad, but I personally enjoy to see someone looking little more muscular and having nice curves on his/her body. As long as you are a beginner with going to the gym, I would advise to try doing exercise with weights for building some muscle mass, even if your main purpose is losing weight. That means to use weights as heavy as you can do 8 repetitions in 4 sets per exercise.

In case we get sick and have a cold, it is recommendable to stop running or exercising for that week. As much as we have that iron will to get rid of the adipose layer, during the time when we have a cold, our system will use all the nutrients and proteins in our body to serve for healing. Then, it does not make sense to run. The same think it happens when a female has her monthly period. Even if she might feel fine and strong for those days, the process of losing weight does not work the same as before. The hormonal changes do not allow her to lose adipose layer during those 4 days even if running. Additionally, during those days a female seems to have a higher appetite for food. Do not worry! That food will not form fat for those 4 days, even if not exercising. That food is going towards the body and blood recovery because a quantity of blood gets lost and a new blood forms to replace it.

As I have also mentioned in the gaining weight chapter, losing weight has a close relationship with carbohydrates. Try eating complex carbohydrates at all times and avoid simple ones. The simple carbs raise the insulin level too fast and soon after, they decrease it even lower than it was initially. That means we are feeling tired soon after we had that boost of energy. If we do not have so much toxins in the body, in order to feel energized all the time, we need to eat complex carbs or simple carbs with a low glycemic index. A good source of carbohydrates is brown or white rice, potatoes (even if they act like simple carbs), whole cereals with no sugar added in composition, whole wheat pasta and others. Fruits and vegetables are simple carbs, too but they act like complex carbs. They are good to be eaten when trying to lose weight but not into a huge quantity. They do not raise the insulin so quickly because they have a low glycemic index. A good combination would be carbs with vegetables or proteins with vegetables. Fruits are good to be eaten by themselves at a separate time. The carbohydrates are digestible different as the way proteins get digested. It is recommended the proteins to be consumed at a different time than the carbohydrates. This is advisable but not mandatory for losing fat. As much as we separate the groups of food one of the other and stop eating before feeling full to the stomach, we should see a tremendous change to our shape.

After couple of months when our system will get used to the diet, we may notice our body gets stuck and it does not want to lose fat anymore. It stops responding to the diet. That is the moment when we have to do a change. We may do a change in the way we exercise or a change in our diet. For example, we can get rid of the salt in our diet. When we do not add salt on our food, we can lose fat easier. The salt retains water in our system and also toxins with it. When the water does not flow quick and it does not pass through the body to cleanse, it will be harder for the body to get rid of the fat. Moreover, the salt accelerates the intestinal absorption of the glucose.

On another hand, when we stop adding salt on our food, we need to take additional salts. There are certain salts, minerals that we cannot avoid to use. For example, we could do very bad muscle cramps if we do not have enough calcium or magnesium in our system. In this case a cramp could come anytime we lay down, relaxing in the bed or lifting weights at the gym. In addition, we have to be careful with stop eating salt when we suffer of low blood pressure.

We know that – you are what you eat. If you eat cow

meat, you will be a cow. If you eat only vegetables, you will become a vegetable. Better cow than vegetable! Eating a pork, you are dirty inside like a pig because pork meat indeed is the most toxic meat. Over all, it is good to eat little bit from everything and not only one type of food. Surely, we have to rely more on chicken, fish, see food, cow (being a red meat, it does not digest so easy but it has its benefits when eaten in small quantities at a time), nuts, milk products, eggs as sources of proteins.

It is very helpful to take some nutritional supplements for losing fat. I was mentioning earlier about the amino acid L-Carnitine which stimulates the brain and it is also very helpful for the losing fat process. When used 500 mg, 1000 mg or 2000 mg at one time before exercise, L-Carnitine transforms a higher amount of fat into source of energy. A low dose of 500 mg is effective as well. This way the energy comes more from the fat and it does not come so much from the muscles. It helps at maintaining the muscle mass. L-Carnitine makes you sweat more when doing aerobic exercise and you will start to lose fat earlier during your running session.

Here is a very important role that omega 3 has or the combination of omega 3, 6 and 9. You can find these in fish oil, flex oil or other. They are the good fats. These bring a tremendous help in the fat loss procedure. It is more effective when you take these supplements before a fatty meal. This way the fat from the food will slide easier outside the body. Attention! Too much fat is bad for us but it is not so dangerous as the carbohydrates are, related to the fat loss procedure. When we choose to do a mistake once in a while eating a piece of bad food, we may better choose fat than carbs. Anyway, this does not mean we should consume lots of bad fats too often.

Mentioning about mistakes, yes, we may do mistakes in our diet one time per week. Attention! I meant one time per week, not one day per week. The one per week mistake means, whatever our body asks for, whatever we crave to eat for. This usually it refers to a simple carb. It could be a cake, a greasy food or fried food, a pastry, chocolate or any "unpermitted" food.

Doing a mistake one time per week, it will just boost the metabolism. It will not trigger any sign for your body to start gathering deposits yet. By dieting, your system gets depleted of glycogen. When doing that eating mistake, the system will fill out those glycogen needs but it will not deposit fat. Otherwise, by doing the mistake too long as a whole day mistake, your body will need another 2 days after that to get rid of that accumulated glucose and only after 2 days, you will continue to start losing fat again. That means, you are losing 3 days from the losing fat procedure. Some people choose to do that mistake once per 2 weeks or never. That is good but not necessarily healthy. When you deplete your body completely of simple carbs for a long period of time or after 2 months of doing so, the tendency of quit dieting is stronger.

When doing severe diets, it is hard to keep them for the whole life. A very severe diet has pluses and minuses. It is true, it helps you faster to look good, but it will decrease your metabolism and you will see yourself in the situation when your body will need more and more severe diets year after year. You will have to get rid of more and more type of foods from your eating style and ingest less and less food quantity. That will be harder and harder, year after year because your cravings will stay the same. It is good to keep your diets as less severe as possible. For competitors is different because they need to reach the minimum adipose layer possible. Now, if you start your diet from a point when you have a lot of fat, it will take a lot of time to lose all your unwanted fat by having less severe diets. That is why, the idea of a strict diet including a mistake time to time with it, is not bad.

I have heard people trying diets with no food at all or too little bit of food. Firstly, this is not healthy. We will create problems for our stomach and a lot of other issues for our system if we do not eat. Unless we are close to be saints or very close by God, we cannot survive without food. Even those type of people who are monks or similar to one, they do not keep the fasten forever. A regular human who leaves a regular life would not be healthy by not eating from all the food categories and when not drinking enough liquid. Moreover, a regular person who does exercise, needs some additional nutritional supplements to complete his daily meals. We are not able to digest a large quantity of regular food in order to have the complete nutrition the body needs throughout the day. Plus, the protein in the regular food comes with fat. It does not come separately. When you need to lose fat but remain with muscle mass or even to increase it, you should take certain additional supplements. When working to your fat loss, it is advisable to take amino acids only or protein powder containing 80% to 100% protein. For a better absorption, it is helpful to use them on empty stomach.

Some people wonder: "I do not eat much during the day. I only eat 2 or 3 times per day and I do not consume a big quantity of food. Why do I still gain weight?" Well, the answer is within the question. You gain weight **because you do not eat**. Do not forget to eat often but little. Even if a meal contains an apple only, it is very important that meal still exists. It is imperative to do eat and the type of food you eat! Eating only 2 croissants for a whole day thinking we need to eat less, it is totally wrong. You are not doing anything else than making your system hungry. When somebody is hungry, it will crave for more food. Those croissants will go straight into fat deposits for two reasons: they are a too little amount of food for a whole day – the body saves up and they are carbohydrates - they are converted faster into fat than even saturated fat into fat.

Do not eat fried food – is another important thing you have to keep in mind when trying to lose weight. Any oil when fried, it is not healthy more or less. If we wanted to eat once in a while a fried food, it would be a good idea to use oils which burn at a higher temperature, over 200 degrees Celsius. These are oils who produce less toxins when we use them to fry the food with. Less toxins means a faster fat loss procedure.

During a diet it is advisable to eat most of the daily carbohydrates in the first part of the day. For a strict diet we should eat all our carbs before 3 pm. They give the energy necessary for the day. In the evening we do not need energy. Our body will soon lay down and rest. When sleeping, the system does not need a lot of energy. The metabolism gets slower. During the night our body uses the nutrients and glycogen that he already has. The moment we wake up, the system is depleted. He asks us for food and liquid supplies. In the morning our system asks mainly for carbohydrates because he needs energy. He will absorb right away whatever we give him and he will not form fat deposits out of the breakfast meal. Breakfast is the most important meal of the day.

We must never skip it. Theoretically, we could eat almost any type of food at the first meal of the day. It also depends of the type of activities we do and the volume of physical work throughout the day. You may eat any combination of proteins with carbs and veggies or only carbs and vegetables. The carbohydrates should not be forgotten. They must be included in the first meal of the day.

It is known that you should keep the breakfast for yourself, share the lunch with friends and dinner give it to the enemies.

For lunch we may still eat a consistent meal. We still need energy for the rest of the day. But, starting with 3 o'clock the carbohydrates should be limited or all avoided. See weight loss eating diets that I composed further down in the book.

When speaking about fruits, it is good to mention that the sugar they contain is called fructose. When using the fructose, we should choose the one which is naturally extracted and not the processed artificially one. During a diet we may use fructose to mix in our coffee, for example. But the fructose usage should be limited. The natural fructose gives energy slow but it does not have the same quality like a complex carbohydrate.

It is imperative the fibers usage within our fat loss process! Without them, it would be almost impossible to lose fat. They clean very good our colon releasing the toxins. If we are constipated, the intestines get clogged up and that impacts all the processes in our system. The buttock is the boss. When he is stressed out, everybody else get nervous. In this case, all the other organs become upset. Fibers are the laborers who usually resolve the situation. Vegetables, fruits and cereals contain fibers. You may eat as many vegetables as you want per day. Even if they contain their sugar called "leguminoza", veggies can be eaten a lot. They do not offer you fat deposits.

There are certain fruits which should be limited as grapes, ripe bananas, honey melon or pineapple. They have a higher glycemic index. Their fructose is assimilated quicker.

Here we may also speak about the dry fruits. They are good to be eaten during the diet but we have to limit them. They help our digestion, cover our potassium and magnesium needs and give energy. But their fructose concentration is high. We have to be careful with them. Sometimes we find them covered in a lot of sugar which is unreasonable added. They need to be completely avoided when they are in that form.

It is sad that certain types of milk contain sugar as preservative. We have to be careful and avoid them. As well as sweet yogurts or sweet cheese. Even many types of sausages contain sugar. That is really disgusting for me but unfortunately, many people find that a good regular taste. This is the way they have grown up, like this they are used to and it seems very natural and tasty for them. It is incredible! We need to take our time and search between the items in the store, hoping we find healthy products. In order to lose fat, you need to be very attentive what you buy and read the labels carefully. Moreover, some products might not even have written on the label that they contain sugar or sugars. Then, why do they taste sweet ???

For a nice shape development and for having the necessary nutrients, we should also use nutritional supplements. Here we have to be careful and read the labels as well. Many nutritional supplements contain sugars with high glycemic index. It is recommended to avoid supplements with a lot of carbs. Some of them contain dextrose or glucose who makes you to gain a not qualitative weight and accumulate unwanted fat. Protein bars are not recommended to be consumed when we want to lose fat. Usually they have in composition a lot of simple carbohydrates along with proteins. They are only good for gaining both together muscular mass and fat. Unless we do the keto diet but eat a protein bar after our heavy lifting workout only, otherwise we would gain fat because of them.

Trying to lose weight without exercising is possible but not recommended. Moreover, in order to have a nice shape we should do both aerobic and anaerobic movements. If we do not exercise, when we keep a diet, the results will be slower and we will never look perfect. Even if we just run but not lifting weights, our shape will not be as perfect as we are dreaming to be and we will not be able to get rid of the all unwanted fat. The little bit of muscles we build, they will help us in the losing fat process and give us a nicer shape. To conclude, if we do not exercise at all, we may lose some fat by dieting only but, the little bit of muscle fibers we have on our body will not be developed. They will get atrophied and soft with no strength. The muscle tissue will be looking dropped and not attractive.

Chapter 4

Gain Weight Diets

There are people who wish to gain weight and they wonder how they can get some fat on them. They need to know that adding fat is not a good solution in order to stay healthy. What they need to add is muscle mass but not much fat. It is always a nicer shape when our mass is formed out of muscles and hard meat, than of fat and jelly that is hanging around.

In order to gain muscle mass, we need to eat more than when is the time to focus on the losing fat process. It is important not to gain too much fat during the gaining muscle mass process. It will be harder for us to lose that fat during the following diet period.

Unfortunately, we will lose some muscle mass too, if we have a too strict diet. When we focus on gaining muscles firstly, we may use certain types of complex carbs as white potatoes or corn which behave like simple carbs because they have a higher glycemic index. Or, we may use white rice which is a simple carbohydrate but a good one for bodybuilders or for those who wish to gain weight because it gives the energy slower.   These are only few examples of tricks we could use for gaining muscle mass without adding too much adipose layer. When we focus on gaining weight, we may even use fried food time to time like fried plantains, but do not exaggerate with it. Otherwise you may form too much toxins. Use the proper cooking oils. The food that we are allowed or not to eat, depends very much of our metabolism and our genetics. When one's metabolism is very fast, he may do more mistakes in his eating habits. But, it is important for everybody, like a general rule, do not eat chaotic without your personal health principles. Do not eat meal after meal with less than 2 hours break in between. Allow your system to digest all the food it already has inside and have an empty stomach, before you introduce more food in it. Otherwise, your system will become very confused. It will be overwhelmed. It will not have time to digest the nutrients and the organs will get stuck with way too much work to do.

In the past, during the off season, bodybuilders let

themselves to gain a lot of fat, too. They said they can have more strength and they could build more muscle this way underneath. This concept has also few disadvantages. In the last few years, bodybuilders avoid this concept and try to maintain a limit of the adipose layer during the off season, too, and avoid the protruding belly. This option seems much clever and should be followed from now on!

There are 3 body types. Each of them has a different metabolism. The ectomorph body type has a faster metabolism. For this type of individual, we need to adapt the gaining weight diet in order to be able to have a lucrative growth. He need to eat more carbs and proteins because his burnings are high. His body has the ability to lose fat easy but he may struggle with gaining muscle mass. This person is allowed to do more mistakes in his eating habits but it will help not to exaggerate with candies, cakes or bad fats anyway. He would gain more qualitative muscle mass by using 80% permitted food and he will have more effective workouts by maintaining a balanced diet. What he has to do is to raise the quantity of the permitted food and he should have a qualitative growth.

The followings are gaining weight diets for **male body types.**

The first one will be the description for a **male ectomorph**. He has to adapt the food quantities by his body weight. Anyway, do not enlarge the stomach and intestines by eating way too much, until you get sick, just for the wish of becoming big. Unfortunately, there are these type of mentalities, too. I have seen those bodybuilders with 4 plates in front of them at one meal. In response to that, their intestines enlarge and they develop a thick waist. They are able to become ripped with no adipose layer on top and with very defined pack abs but, they cannot do anything to help their protruding stomach.

Ectomorph gain weight diet:
<u>Monday</u>
6:30 am – protein powder shake (30 – 50% protein)
7 am – corn meal with 5 eggs (2 yolks only) and cheese + orange juice
9 am – protein bar (>=20 grams protein)
10 am – potatoes salad with chicken (300 grams) and veggies and oil
12 pm – amino acids
1 pm – white rice + steak 200 grams + pickles
4 pm – fruit salad + honey + nuts
workout (lifting weights only)
6 pm – whey protein shake (50 – 70% protein)
7 pm – 2 chicken legs + rice + beans + green salad

(lettuce)
9 pm – amino acids
10 pm – 5 egg whites + avocado + radish
3 am – amino acids

Tuesday
6: 30 am – protein powder shake (30 - 50% protein)
7 am – 6 eggs omelet with spinach and cheese (2 yolks only) + 2 slices bread and butter + barley with milk
9 am – protein bar (>=20 grams protein)
10 am – yams(not sweet potatoes) + beef + black beans
12 pm – amino acids
1 pm – yams + chicken + peas, carrots, avocado oil
4 pm – oatmeal + banana + blueberry + raisins + honey
workout (lifting weights + running)
6 pm – protein shake (50% protein)
7 pm - quinoa salad with chicken, peas, carrots, avocado oil
10 pm – casein protein shake (70 – 80% protein)
3 am – amino acids

Wednesday
6:30 am – protein powder shake (30-50% protein)
7 am – 6 eggs omelet with ham (2 yolks only) + cheese + 2 slices bread with butter + 2 cups milk with honey
9 am – protein bar (>=20 grams protein)
10 am – fried plantains + chicken leg + green salad

12 pm – fruits (any type)
1 pm - white pasta + shrimp + mixed veggies + lentils
3 pm – workout (weight lifting only)
4 pm – protein shake (50% protein)
5 pm – pasta + shrimp + veggies (the left over) + lentils
7 pm – amino acids
8 pm – nuts + plain kefir (3/4 liter) + dried fruits
10 pm – casein protein shake
3 am – amino acids

Thursday
6:30 am – protein shake (50% protein)
7 am – 6 eggs (3 yolks only) + plantains + asparagus + orange juice
9 am – protein bar (>=20 grams protein)
10 am – protein shake
10:30 am – fruits (peaches or mangos)
12 pm – sweet potatoes + beef (200 grams) + black beans + beet
3 pm – potatoes + beef (left over) + black beans + pickles
6 pm – scallop + quinoa + tomato sauce
9 pm – scallop + tomato sauce
10 pm – amino acids
3 am – amino acids

Friday
6:30 am - protein shake

7 am – fish sticks(10) + white rice + cornmeal with milk
10 am – fruit salad + nuts + honey
12 pm – protein bar (>=20 grams protein)
1 pm – yams + baked chicken + green beans + broccoli
3 pm – workout (weight lifting only)
4 pm – protein shake
5 pm – yams + baked chicken (left over) + greens
7 pm – amino acids
8 pm – ham + kefir (1 liter) + nuts
10 pm – casein protein shake
3 pm – amino acids

Saturday

6:30 am – protein shake (30-50% protein)
7 am – 3 eggs + 1 slice bread + peanut butter + jelly + 2 cups whole milk
9 am – protein bar
10 am – sweet potatoes + beef + green leaves
1 pm – workout (weight lifting only)
2 pm – protein shake (30 – 50% protein)
3 pm – cornmeal + whole milk kefir + dried fruits
4 pm – fruits + honey
6 pm – amino acids
7 pm – beef + veggies (the left over) + potatoes
10 pm – casein protein powder
3 am – amino acids

<u>Sunday</u>
sleep
9 am – protein shake
10 am – potato salad + chicken with skin + peas + hot chocolate milk
1 pm – 1 slice cake (or your favorite unpermitted desert)
4 pm – omelet + mushrooms + ham + spinach + potatoes
6 pm – amino acids
7 pm – chicken + peas + spinach + potatoes
10 pm – protein shake
3 am – amino acids

In order to grow we must eat like a baby, once per 2,5 hours or 3 hours. A baby is also eating during the night to make sure he does not lose weight and he keeps growing. The same way we have to do, too. We need sleep and often meals. When we wake up during the night, take a quick portion of amino to keep growing. The amino acids are the compounds of the protein. Your body does not need to put much effort in decomposing them. You will be able to continue your restful sleep. Some people choose to wake up 2 times per night to take twice amino acids and go back to sleep right away. If this schedule makes you tired and you do not fall asleep right away, it is better to continue sleeping. Only a good sleep helps the growth.

Another body type is the mesomorph one. This is a type as the majority of us have. A mesomorph person is one who cannot gain weight and lose fat very easy but not very hard either. This is a combination of the other 2 body types: ectomorph and endomorph. It is like an average between the two. Even if it is off season and the gaining mass period, this individual should not eat gravy or bad fats. When for an ectomorph type, it might be permitted to do such a mistake once in a while, this would do really bad for a mesomorph or endomorph one. A fried (bad or good) fat is worse than a bad fat which has not been fried. It makes us sluggish and this will have a negative impact over our workouts.

Mesomorph gain weight diet:
Monday
6: 30 am – protein powder shake (50% protein)
7 am – 3 eggs omelet with spinach and cheese (2 yolks only) + 1 slice toast bread and butter + barley with milk
9 am – protein bar (>=20 grams protein)
10 am - yams(not sweet potatoes) + beef + black beans
12 pm – amino acids
1 pm – yams + chicken, peas, carrots, avocado oil (200 grams)
4 pm – oatmeal + banana + blueberry + raisins + honey
workout (lifting weights only)
7 pm - quinoa salad with chicken, peas, carrots, avocado

oil
10 pm – casein protein shake (70 – 80% protein)
3 am – amino acids

<u>Tuesday</u>
6:30 am – protein shake (50% protein)
7 am – oatmeal with 3 eggs (2 yolks only) + cheese +
orange
juice (no sugar)
9 am – protein bar (>=20 grams protein)
10 am – potatoes salad with chicken (200 grams) +
veggies with olive oil
1 pm – brown rice + steak (200 grams) + pickles
3 pm – amino acids
4 pm – fruit salad + nuts + low fat sour cream
workout(weight lifting only)
6 pm – whey protein concentrate (50% protein)
7 pm – 1 chicken leg + quinoa + beans + green salad
10 pm – 3 egg whites + avocado + radish
3 am – amino acids

<u>Wednesday</u>
6:30 am – protein shake + 1 banana (50% protein)
running
7 am – 3 eggs omelet with ham (2 yolks only) + cheese +
1 slice toast bread and butter + 1 cup milk with 1 spoon
honey

10 am – boiled plantains + chicken leg + green salad
1 pm – whole wheat pasta + shrimp + green salad
3 pm – amino acids
4 pm – whole wheat pasta + shrimp + veggies
7 pm – nuts + plain kefir (2 cups)
10 pm – casein protein concentrate (80 % protein)
3 pm – amino acids

Thursday

6:30 am – protein concentrate (50% protein)
7 am – whole wheat pasta + 3 eggs + cheese + 1 cup milk and 1 spoon honey
10 am – 1 peach
10:30 am – protein bar (>=20 grams protein)
1 pm - yam + fish (200 grams) + broccoli
4 pm – yam + fish + broccoli
5 pm - workout (weight lifting only)
6 pm – whey protein concentrate
7 pm – chicken + quinoa + pickles (no sugar)
10 pm – casein protein concentrate (80% protein)
3 pm – amino acids

Friday

6: 30 am – protein shake (50% protein)
7 am – 3 eggs omelet (max. 2 yolks) + mushrooms and ham + 1 toast slice white bread + radish + 1 cup milk and 1 spoon honey

9 am – protein bar (>=20 grams protein)
10 am – white rice + boiled beef + pickles
1 pm – greens juice (spinach, basil, apple, etc.)
4 pm – sea food saute + white rice + tomatoes
workout (lifting weights only)
6 pm – whey protein concentrate
7 pm – sea food + quinoa + tomatoes + peas
10 pm – 3 egg whites + peas
3 pm – amino acids

Saturday
6:30 am – amino acids
running
7 am – barley + berries + banana + low fat sour cream
10 am – 3 corn cubs
1 pm – whey protein concentrate
4 pm – chicken + quinoa + bean pods
7 pm – chicken + quinoa + bean pods
10 pm – casein protein concentrate (80% protein)
3 pm - amino acids

Sunday
sleep
9 am – protein shake
10 am – 3 eggs + 1 slice toast bread + carrots
1 pm – 1 slice cake (or your favorite desert)
4 pm – beef + rice + green juice

7 pm – beef + rice + green juice
10 pm – nuts + kefir (2 cups)
3 am – amino acids

   The third type of human body is the endomorph one. This individual encounters issues during the losing fat process and it is harder for him to get ripped. He builds muscle mass quite easy but it is hard for him to uncover it and show it. It is advisable for him to limit the carbs with high glycemic index in the off season as well. This way he will not have such a head ache with losing fat in season. This way only, he will be able to have the same diet type before competition, as the diet type of a mesomorph competitor who was not so careful with the carbs in his off season. Including restrictions during his diet, the endomorph individual will also be healthier all year long. This last idea applies to the all 3 body types.

<u>Endomorph gain weight diet:</u>
<u>Monday</u>
6:30 am – amino acids
7 am – 3 eggs (1 yolk) + ham + oatmeal + 1 cup milk
9 am – amino acids
10 am - fruit salad + nuts + low fat sour cream
1 pm – protein bar (>=20 grams protein)
4 pm – chicken + rice + beans + green salad
workout (weight lifting + running)

6 pm – whey protein concentrate (50% protein)
7 pm – 1 chicken legs + beans + green salad
10 pm – amino acids
3 pm – amino acids

Tuesday

6: 30 am – amino acids
7 am – 3 eggs omelet + mushrooms + 1 slice toast whole wheat bread
9 am – amino acids
10 am – fruits (any type)
1 pm – chicken thigh + quinoa + veggies
4 pm – rice + steak (100 grams) + bean pods + beet workout (weight lifting only)
6 pm – whey protein concentrate (50% protein)
7 pm – beef + bean pods
10 pm – amino acids
3 pm – amino acids

Wednesday

6:30 am – amino acids
7 am – 3 eggs (2 yolks) + cheese + 1 slice toast whole wheat bread
9 am – amino acids
10 am – 2 corn cubs + 1 banana
12 pm – amino acids
1 pm – fish + boiled carrots + whole wheat pasta

running
4 pm – protein shake (50% protein)
7 pm – fish + veggies
10 pm – nuts + kefir (1 cup)
3 pm - amino acids

Thursday
6:30 am – amino acids
7 am - fruits
9 am - amino acids
10 am – potato salad (potato, boiled eggs, olives, onion, oil)
1 pm – brown rice + beef + green salad (lettuce) + olive oil
4 pm – protein bar
workout
6 pm – protein shake (50% protein)
7 pm – beef + lettuce + olive oil
10 pm – amino acids
3 pm amino acids

Friday
6:30 am – protein shake (50% protein)
7 am – milk + cereals(no sugar), 2 eggs (1 yolk) omelet + ham + spinach + rice cake
9 am – amino acids
10 am - fruits + nuts + sour cream

1 pm – pasta + extra virgin olive oil + veggies saute (ex: pepper, eggplant, carrot, squash)
4 pm – fish + pasta + tomato sauce
workout (weight lifting only)
6 pm – amino acids
7 pm – fish + broccoli
10 pm – 3 egg whites + broccoli
3 am – amino acids

Saturday
6:30 am – amino acids
running
7 am – greens juice + pasta + extra virgin olive oil (or similar)
10 am – fruits
12 pm – amino acids
1 pm – chicken + whole wheat pasta + squash + bell pepper
4 pm – chicken + quinoa + veggies
7 pm – chicken + kefir
10 pm – protein casein shake (>70% protein)
3 am – amino acids

Sunday
sleep
9 am – greens juice (spinach + apple + etc.)
10 am – eggs + 1 slice toast bread + tomato and

cucumber salad

12 pm – amino acids

1 pm – 1 slice cake (or your favorite desert)

4 pm – beef + rice + veggies

6 pm – amino acids

7 pm – beef + veggies

10 pm – casein protein shake (80% protein)

3 am – amino acids

As you see, the diet for endomorphs is made with brown rice or whole pasta because these foods have a low glycemic index and an endomorph type may gain fat quite easier. Do not forget, in case your stomach gets bloated or in pain because of the hard digestion of these carbs, skip to the regular white rice and white pasta and reduce the quantity.

Gaining weight for a female is little bit different than gaining weight for the male. She has different types of hormones and she may metabolize the food slower than a male. A female usually has less weight, so she has to eat less food. There are the same 3 body types as for the males, but from the diet point of view, the natural female may lower the food quantities mentioned above. Otherwise, she may gain easier adipose layer underneath her skin. Even if the female wishes to gain muscle mass and she needs to eat more for this to happen, she does not have to force herself to eat big amounts of food at only one meal. She will enlarge her stomach and appetite. She will feel hungrier as the time passes and she will ask for more food. This and the fact that she might keep too strict diets during the season time, it will affect her metabolism. She will need to have more restrictions in her diets as the time passes, after few years of keep doing this routine.

A female of an average weight should never eat the food quantities of an ectomorph male. When she wishes to gain muscle mass, she may eat the types of food that an ectomorph male eats. She may eat similar as an endomorph male in terms of quantities.

The estrogen a female has, it does not allow her to build so easy muscle mass as a male or to lose fat so easy as a male does. The same way it happens for a male who has more estrogen. It is harder for him to lose fat or gain muscles easy. That is why we have to compensate this unfortunate genetic and help our body by developing a natural anabolic effect. This anabolism may be gained by eating healthy food as a semi diet and by exercise regularly.

Here is an example of gaining weight diet for one female of an average weight (**not** for a professional bodybuilder). It is advisable to have only one larger meal per day, preferably before 4 pm. The rest of the meals should not overfill the stomach.

Example:
6:30 am – protein shake (50% protein)
7 am – 3 eggs (2 yolks) + ham + tomato + 1 slice toast bread
10 am – oatmeal flakes + raisins + banana + kefir
12 pm – amino acids
1 pm – rice + beef (100 grams) + homemade pickles, 1 cup green juice (spinach, apple, basil leaves)
4 pm – rice + beef (50 grams) + veggies
workout
6 pm – protein shake (50% protein)
7 pm – fish (100 grams) + asparagus + homemade tomato sauce (tomato, garlic, thyme)
10 am – 2 egg whites + nuts + homemade tomato sauce

When this is too much food for a certain female, she may skip one of the meals. She may replace it with amino acids only, making sure the body keeps receiving time to time nutrition. As we can see, the diet contains food from all categories. You only have to add the other necessary supplements described in the other chapters as Omega 3, vitamins, minerals and the very effective amino acids or the protein powder. The protein concentrate is present only 2 times per day, at the times with maximum absorption, because it has 50% carbohydrate. It exists the risk of gaining too much adipose layer on top of the muscle mass when this is taken other times of the day. During the gaining weight period, the protein powder that contains some carbs too, is very effective for muscular growth.

All the body types should take some supplements before and after the exercise routine. Along with the protein supplements, we should not forget the vitamins and minerals. Without them we cannot be healthy when we do exercise regularly.

As you see for the endomorph type, the amount of food is reduced and the carbs with high glycemic index are limited because this individual has slow burnings. The amount of amino acids is increased and the protein powder that contains carbs is limited, to make sure he does not gain way too much fat besides muscles. The fat layer should be kept under control at any time. Everybody should realize how his own system does respond. If he feels he does not have enough energy, he may increase the supplementation in this matter or the complex carbs quantity.

All these processes happen for a natural body. When people use additional testosterone, the things stay different. The body may get both upset and happy. The liver gets enlarged right away but, it comes back to its initial measurements once you stop using the substance. It is risky to take testosterone from outside. It is a chemical which behaves as any other chemical in the human body. It forms toxins. This is why, certain testosterone supplements trigger pimples on the skin as a reaction of the body who wants to get rid of those toxins. When people take it for a long time and in big quantities, it may reduce their own natural testosterone production. That is a side effect that makes the body to increase his estrogen which is very bad for a man who wants to compete and not only. It may trigger "bitch tits" at males and the adipose layer may develop easier on the body. It is even worse for kids under 18 years old. Their natural testosterone is just forming. Taking testosterone at a such young age, it inhibits even worse the own natural testosterone to develop.

Many times, we may find people belonging to two categories in the same time. As an example, a mesomorph may have certain features from an endomorph type. Moreover, people have different weight and different preferences or sensitivities for certain foods. We cannot force ourselves to eat the same. That is why we need to adjust the diet for each separate individual. The examples above give an idea of healthy food and the necessity of having more meals per day as well as it teaches how to combine the food categories and not bring a confusion to your own body system. When you are young, your digestive system may work well and the metabolism may be faster. For an older person the things may change. His body may process the food slower. He may gain fat easier. He should be more careful when trying to build muscle mass by eating a huge food quantity. His body might clog up with too many acidic proteins. Because an old person is not able to build muscles at the same level as the young one, he should not eat the same quantity hoping he will grow big muscle mass. A male starts to lose his natural testosterone after 45 years old. This impacts the ability to increase his muscle mass on a natural way. By then, a male should have already build a lot of muscles. Then, he could maintain a nice shape easier before 55 years old when he will see another difference in his looks and the skin quality. Of course, this differs from one person to another. It depends of his stress level and his active or sedentary life.

Chapter 5

Weight Loss Diets

Everybody should create his personal eating habits and make changes after his personal needs and body reactions. Every one of us feels different, his body reacts different than his friends or colleague's body. Unfortunately, not all of us have the necessary time to keep track about all the processes our system goes through and not all of us have the mind open for a thorough thinking in this direction. That is why sometimes we need the help of a health care professional specialized in diets or a nutritionist as well as a general health practitioner for being up to date with our blood levels. Strict diets could be very dangerous and harmful for our system, we could lose too many vitamins, minerals and become weak. Not having a balanced diet and proper vitamins or supplementation, it may increase the risk of illness or even death. Even if we may keep under control our health, sometimes our body could surprise us with its reaction to certain substances or food combinations. Different environments we are exposed to, the stress or food could affect us in an unexpected way at different times. Medicine evolves, every day researchers may find different cures or substances that could help us. We might need to avoid certain medicine or compounds, but we do not know about that at the present time. We do not know everything, even if we think we know.

This chapter offers information about certain foods that help us to lose weight when eaten at the right time of the day. Do not have to follow in particular one of the diets listed below. You have to accommodate them after your personal needs and body reactions. The best food for the system is the one cooked at home. Who does not know to cook, he has to start learning it. We may just resume to simple food which can be cooked easy without complicate recipes. These ones are digested easier by our body anyway and the system would enjoy them better.

There are 2 types of slim persons. One may look thin

but soft with no curved shapes. Someone else is fit with nice curves and her/his body has a hard meat which does not shake at touch. Which one would you like to be?

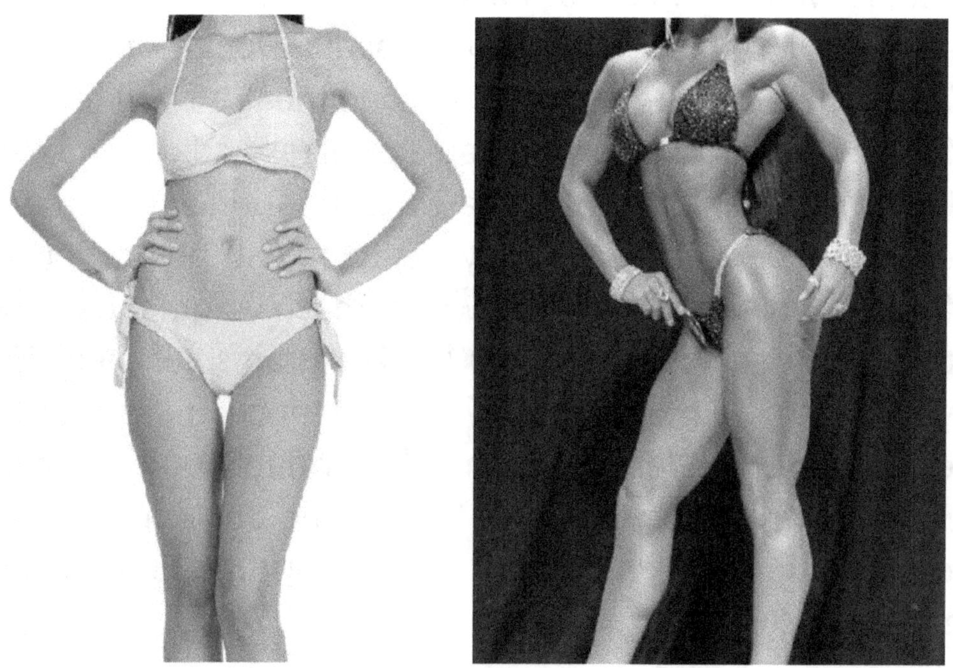

Bellow you find examples of **diets for people who exercise** as well. Without cardio and weight lifting, the body is sluggish and it would be harder to reach the goal. When we want to lose fat, we have to eat at one meal as much as we do not feel full in the stomach yet. Even if our craving would push us to take more, please stop before feeling full in order to lose adipose layer. We should start eating again only when our stomach feels empty for at least 15 minutes and if only at least 2 hours passed by. For losing fat, we may even wait for 4 hours before starting to eat again. If we did a mistake and eat too much at one time (ex: a too big piece of steak), we should wait for hours, as long as our stomach needs to get empty, before starting to eat again. Do not take a break for over 4 hours long between meals. If you feel full because of the portion you eat, please adjust and eat less. Measurements are not always mentioned in these examples because everybody has to adjust the portion for his own weight and his own stomach volume. Usually the meat size has to be of 100 or 200 grams per meal. If you feel that 6 meals per day are too much, make them 5 only. Do not eat less than 5 meals per day! You can pick up meals from the examples bellow and do your own combination but keep the same hour or time for eating them.

Example 1 for one week diet:

<u>Monday</u>
7 am – pure oatmeal flakes + unsweet plain kefir + 20 raisins
10 am – 1 banana
1 pm – brown rice + chicken breast + green salad
4 pm – grated fresh apple and carrot
7 pm – boiled beef + broccoli
10 pm – 2 boiled egg whites + tomato

<u>Tuesday</u>
7 am – 2 eggs + 1 toast bread + lean ham + bell pepper
10 am – 1 mango
1 pm – brown rice + baked fish
4 pm – veggie salad + extra virgin olive oil
7 pm – grilled chicken breast + avocado
10 pm – casein protein powder (90 – 100% protein) + water

<u>Wednesday</u>
7 am – 1 bowl of brown rice + dried fruits (do not over eat)
10 am – grapes (not in large amount)
1 pm – 2 rice cakes + butter + turkey ham + green pepper
4 pm – 2 eggs omelet + mushrooms + tomato
7 pm – veggies + chicken + sesame oil salad
10 pm - amino acids

<u>Thursday</u>
7 am – boiled barley + strawberries + drops of maple syrup
10 am – half grapefruit
1 pm – baked red potatoes + steak
4 pm – grated fresh apple and carrot
7 pm – fish + lots of grilled vegetable mix (squash, green/red pepper, onion, broccoli, etc.)
10 pm – nuts

<u>Friday</u>
7 am – fruit salad (mixed berries, banana, etc.) + nuts + drops of maple syrup
10 am – egg + 1 toast slice bread + cucumber
1 pm – 1 chicken leg with no skin + beans
4 pm – grated fresh apple and carrot
7 pm – grilled shrimp + quinoa + tomatoes + hot pepper
10 pm – protein powder (90-100% protein)

<u>Saturday</u>
7 am – egg omelet with spinach + oatmeal + black coffee
10 am – 1 apple
1 pm – scallop + whole wheat pasta + green beans + fresh tomato sauce (2 tomatoes, thyme, garlic, salt, etc.)
4 pm – 2 rice cakes + lean ham + max. 2 % fat plain yogurt
7 pm – beef + peas + corn
10 pm – amino acids

<u>Sunday</u>
7 am – 2 eggs + 2 rice cake + ham + radish
10 am – 1 orange
1 pm – 1 slice cake (or your favorite unpermitted dessert)
4 pm – red potato + grilled chicken breast + green salad
7 pm – sea food + asparagus
10 pm – nuts

Example 2 for one week diet:

<u>Monday</u>

6:30 am – amino acids

running

7 am – 1 egg + ham + rice cake + milk with cereals

10 am – oatmeal + strawberries

11 am – workout

12 pm – protein shake (80% protein)

1 pm – chicken thigh + brown rice + green salad

4 pm – 1 apple

7 pm – chicken drum stick + beans

10 pm – amino acids

<u>Tuesday</u>

6:30 am – 1/2 grapefruit

running

7 am – 2 eggs + spinach + 1 toast slice whole wheat bread

9 am – workout

10 am – protein shake (80% protein)

11 am – fish + brown rice + beans pods

1 pm – amino acids

4 pm – grated apple and carrot

7 pm – fish (left over from earlier) + bean pods

10 pm – 3 boiled egg whites

<u>Wednesday</u>
6:30 am – amino acids
running
7 am – oatmeal + plain unsweetened kefir + slices banana
10 am – 1 corn
1 pm – farmers cheese + couple dried fruits (no sugar added)
4 pm – boiled beef + green peas
running (optional)
7 pm – boiled beef + green peas (left over)
10 pm - nuts

<u>Thursday</u>
6:30 am – ½ grapefruit
running
7 am – farmers cheese + dried fruits + banana
10 am – 2 boiled eggs + bell pepper
1pm – steamed shrimp + whole wheat pasta + handmade tomatoes sauce
3 pm – workout
4 pm – protein shake (80% protein)
4:30 pm - nuts
7 pm – shrimp + handmade tomatoes sauce (left over)
10 pm – 1 cup unsweetened plain kefir

<u>Friday</u>
6:30 am – amino acids
running
7 am – whole grain unsweetened cereals + milk
10 am – 1 cup blended greens (steamed spinach, 1 apple, fresh basil leaves) + 2 boiled eggs
1 pm – chicken thigh + small red potato + beet
3 pm – workout
4 pm – protein shake (80% protein)
4:30 pm – nuts
6 pm – chicken(left over or not) + salad (cucumber + tomato)
9 pm – farmers cheese + bell pepper

<u>Saturday</u>
6:30 am – 1 banana
running
7 am – kefir + cereals
10 am – 1 corn
1 pm – calamari saute + quinoa + veggies
4 pm – cheese + tomatoes
7 pm – calamari saute (left over) + veggies
running (optional)
10 pm – amino acids

<u>Sunday</u>
7 am – fruit salad

10 am – 2 eggs + quinoa + radish
1 pm – slice of cake (or your favorite unpermitted food)
4 pm – chicken breast + quinoa + green salad
7 pm – farmers cheese + sour cream
10 pm – chicken breast + green salad

Attention! All these diets and exercise are made for people who are perfectly healthy. Ask a health care professional before any experiment you do. With so many running sessions and weight lifting, you need to have a healthy heart and joints and keep in touch with your doctor for regular visits. Listen to your symptoms and have everything under control!

The weight loss diets recommend eating whole cereals, whole rice or whole wheat pasta. Do not forget that the whole cereals digest harder. Certain people may experience stomach pain and bloated tummy as soon as they eat whole wheat or other whole cereals. This is because they may form too much acid in their tummy to break them down and the stomach struggles little bit to digest them. Additionally, many people may be sensitive to gluten and they do not know. Even if the whole cereals have a lower glycemic index, fact that makes them good for a fat loss diet, some people cannot digest them easy and it makes them to better avoid eating brown rice or brown pasta and whole wheat bread.

Do not forget: never fill your stomach all the way! Use small meals! Otherwise, we still need to eat enough and diverse food for our body to be healthy. Also, people who do strenuous activity, mostly with their brain all day long or at least 8 hours pe day, they need a lot of energy to focus. Without food supply, our system cannot function. We need to eat even if we want to lose fat! The measurements in grams or ounces need to be adjusted for each individual body weight. Each of us may choose his favorite uncooked oils as dressing or vegetables to use. For the losing fat diets, try not to use oils to fry or bake the food with. Any oil when used for frying is not proper for the fat loss period. These are examples of diets only. Additionally, it depends how large is one's stomach when he starts the diet. After time, he need to eat less and less quantity in order to form a smaller stomach step by step. We cannot shrink the stomach overnight or in couple of weeks only. Eating all of a sudden very little bit, the acid in the stomach might create problems. Then, we cannot continue the losing fat process. Professional or nonprofessional bodybuilders who weight much more than a regular person, eat much more than this. They try to have more grams of protein than these diets comprehend. I am not doing diets for them. They already know their style and nutritional habits. They discover in time what helps and what do not and what changes they should make.

Usually, a natural individual cannot metabolize more than a limit as 100 or at most 200 grams of protein at a time. When one is natural and eat more than his energy consumption daily, his body would develop fat deposits. We may eat little bit more for at most one meal per day only when necessary, for the rest of the meals we must leave a quarter stomach still empty.

In the first 2 weeks of diet, you will feel that your body grows. Yes, the muscles expand. This is a natural reaction of the body when we start eating healthy. Do not worry! The fat does not increase. The fat does not receive the type of food anymore to be able to grow, but the muscles yes!

The example bellow will show separation between the protein and carbohydrates. This is another method of losing fat when your body needs a change, to get rid of the monotony of one certain diet. Additionally, the proteins are digested different than carbs. That means the body will also answer effectively to this kind of diet and the change will be welcome. In order to break down the protein, our body uses acid and for breaking down the carbohydrates, the body needs bases. For this reason, it is a good idea to try eating separate and see if this diet works.

Example 3 for 1 week diet:

<u>Monday</u>
7 am – boiled oatmeal + strawberries
10 am – 1 measure protein shake (80%-100% protein)
1 pm – 1 medium red potato
4 pm – grated apple and carrot
7 pm – chicken breast + green salad
10 pm – chicken breast + asparagus

<u>Tuesday</u>
7 am – fruit salad
10 am – brown rice + broccoli
1 pm – protein shake (80%-100% protein)
4 pm – boiled beef + beans + pickles (homemade, no sugar, no vinegar)
7 pm – boiled beef + beet
10 pm - nuts

<u>Wednesday</u>
7 am – protein shake (70-80% protein)
10 am – whole wheat pasta + homemade tomato sauce (tomato, garlic, salt, basil, etc.)
1 pm – 1 apple
4 pm – baked fish + broccoli
7 pm – baked fish + broccoli
10 pm – farmers cheese + low fat sour cream

Thursday

7 am – brown rice + 20 raisins
10 am – protein shake (80% protein)
1 pm – fruit salad

4 pm – chicken breast (no skin) + avocado
7 pm – chicken breast + steamed spinach
10 pm – cheese + low fat sour cream

Friday

7 am – grapefruit + nuts
10 am – whole wheat pasta + extra virgin olive oil + salt
1 pm – blended vegetable juice (steamed spinach, 1 apple, basil)
4 pm – steak + bean pods
7 pm – steak + bean pods
10 pm – 2 egg whites

Saturday

7 am – oatmeal + banana + strawberries + drops of honey
10 am – protein shake (80% protein)

1 pm – quinoa + black beans
4 pm – shrimp + mixed grilled veggies (squash, eggplant, red pepper, broccoli, etc.)
7 pm – shrimp + veggies
10 pm – 2 egg whites

<u>Sunday</u>
7 am – oatmeal + dried fruits
10 am – fresh fruits
1 pm – 1 slice cake (or your favorite desert)
4 pm – scallop + mixed veggies
7 pm – scallop + veggies
10 pm – protein shake (80-100% protein)

Many people complain about the difficulties with eating diet food while going into an office and spending so many hours out of the house. They would easier go to the cafeteria or cross the street to a quick sandwich place. It is advisable to cook your own meal in order to know what it consists in. This way you can control what you eat. Take cooked food in containers for your lunch break at work, fruits and nutritional supplements. You may even take the left over from your last night dinner and eat the second day at work. In US it is a lot of air conditioning inside the buildings. The food will not go bad. Otherwise, take with you a cooler and every day you may replace the ice plastic inside. There are ways of eating healthy and lose fat or reach your goal. All that you need is a strong will.

Chapter 6

Exercise Types

Everything what helps or gives you happiness, it has its negative impact and it may transform you in a weak person and everything what makes you suffer, it gives you development and abilities to become stronger. Every risk may bring benefits and every benefit brings risks. This is a chapter where you will read about different types of exercises, their risks and benefits. I am going to describe each exercise separately for you to be able to execute it correctly in the gym. Exercising in a correct way is a must! Otherwise, many accidents may happen or a wrong posture of the body may form over time. This could affect the bone structure and implicitly your health.

The posture is also very important during walking or running. If your toes stay inwards at each step, the whole leg will get formed inward starting with the hip. If your toes stay outwards too much at each step, your entire leg will form outwards after a while. The whole structure gets modified this way. It will give you an unhealthy appearance but moreover it will affect your spine. The toes should stay straight when you step or slightly outwards if you wish, but not way too much at the side. Bodybuilders have learned what means a correct posture when doing exercise. But, some people who go to the gym do not keep their back or legs correct when working out. Unfortunately, I have seen lots of those.

There are 2 different types of exercise: aerobic and anaerobic.

Aerobic exercises help to enlarge the thoracic capacity. By doing cardio, we are forced to inhale more air in our lungs and at a higher rate. By breathing in and out consecutively at a steady pace, we bring a higher volume of oxygen in our lungs. This way, we will have healthier cells and blood which help the organs and muscles. Any aerobic exercise is good to be done but running outside is the most effective one. It forces the breathing system to bring a bigger volume of air inside us than any other cardio activity. Running stays as a base for any other sport. A combination of cardio activities would be great, too.

Anaerobic exercises are the ones which are executed without the oxygen presence. In this case, if you exhale too early during your exercise, your body will lose its strength and it will be impossible to end the exercise successfully.

In order to build a proportional body, we need to work out all of the muscle groups on our soft skeleton. By working the upper body only or most of the time, an individual will not develop his lower body. His legs will remain small and his body not proportional. Unfortunately, many males do not like to work their legs. I would say they look like Popeye, the sailor man who eats spinach and his arm biceps is the only muscle who gets big. But this is not true, because Popeye has little bit of muscles to his legs, too. On the other hand, if we work most of the time legs, our upper body will have some tonus, too. The legs consist in a large group of muscles which request a high amount of blood flow when we train them. By working the legs, the blood is pumped in the upper body, too. That maintains also the upper body to stay firm. This does not mean we should work the legs only. But, in case we do not have enough time during a certain week for exercising all our muscle groups, we should put the workout for legs first. In order to develop the legs properly, we should even train them 2 times per week time to time. Being a big group of muscles, they need more work in order to get developed.

Squats (genuflexiuni) are the basic exercise to be done for the legs development. By doing squats we are working the quadriceps and the hamstrings. We may execute this with barbell on the shoulders or with dumbbells. The execution and position of the body should be the same for both. Using the barbell is the most effective way but it also damages your back easier in time because the weight presses the spine vertebras vertically. During the execution, the upper body should lean little bit forward with the shoulders and the glutes backwards. The back should form a little arch. Bending the legs, we get down until our quads are parallel to the ground and come back up. We may stay for a second there in the sitting position but this is not necessary. If we drop our glutes lower than parallel to the ground, the hip area will develop wide. Especially for females, this is not indicated. Even if squat is a basic exercise for legs, it may make your waist area thick when working out for years.

We may do squats to the sliding machine using the incorporated barbell. Those type of squats are safer. The risk of an injury is low but it decreases the benefits, too. The muscle development is limited in comparison with the free barbell squats. Otherwise, during the execution at the squat machine, we may place our feet further or regular, for working the muscles from different angles. Sometimes it is good to exercise this type of squat, too. Some people who lift a lot of weight by squatting, do not go as low as a sitting position. They return back up before getting in that position. This is a theft! By doing so, they steel from themselves. They believe they lift a lot of weight but the exercise is half way done only and their muscle development as well.

Regular deadlift (indreptari) is another basic exercise that is a must for a person who wants a full body development. These types of deadlifts work the body as a whole. They are good for back, shoulders, legs and others. Always execute deadlifts keeping the back straight with a little arch, the same way as doing squats. Keep shoulders and glutes backwards. Legs should be apart with a longer distance between them. Bending the knees, grab with your hands the barbell which is in front of you. Lift the barbell with the legs first and at the half of the distance coming up, use the back to help with lifting the barbell. Pull your shoulders backwards when you are up. Your arms should be always straight. Stop when you are almost vertically straight, but do not come backwards with your back. You may damage your back over time. In power lifting contest, the competitors have to bend backwards at the end of the rep to make sure the referee sees the rep is done all the way. That is the end of the rep for them. Do not do this as a routine. It is very dangerous for the spine. In bodybuilding we have to control the weight all the way back down to the ground. The exercise ends when we are in the initial position only.

Deadlifts with straight legs is a very useful exercise for having nice glutes. For a correct execution we have to stay with the legs straight. Sometimes we may slightly bend the knees. During this exercise we are working the hamstrings and the glutes. Keep your legs close one to the other and the feet parallel. The distance between the feet should be about 10 cm. Grab the barbell in front of you and lift it until you are almost all way up. Do not lean backwards when you are up. The same way as I mentioned for the regular deadlifts, we have to protect our back by not coming up all a way. Going back down to the ground, we have to control the barbell stretching the hamstrings and the glutes. We should drop forward by going with the barbell above the feet and come back. Do not relax when you are standing up at the half of your rep execution, nor between the reps.

Bench press (impins culcat) for chest is the main exercise for the pectoral muscles. We may use different angles to position the bench: inclined forward, backward or straight horizontally. We may work the lower part of the chest by positioning the barbell above the lower part of the chest. This happens easier when the bench is inclined backward and we lay our head lower than the position of the legs. We may work the upper part of the chest by positioning the barbell straight above the upper part of the chest area. Here we may use the bench press positioned horizontally or positioned the way our head is upper than the legs. When we work out the chest in a position with the head higher, the shoulder muscles will be worked, too. When exercising the chest muscles from a horizontally position, we may usually be able to lift heavier weights. During the execution, we should keep our elbows open in both sides of the upper body for working mostly the chest. They should not be placed to touch the body. We must control the arms when our elbows are dropping down. The upper body should remain straight on the bench. Do not arch your back. If you need to arch it, the weight is too heavy for you when your purpose is to build muscle mass. You may keep the feet on the floor or in the air with the knees up. When bringing the barbell downwards to touch your body, the chest needs to be open up. We may touch the chest with the barbell and then lift it back up. We may even strike the barbell against the chest when the weight is heavy to help us lift it up, but this should not be the usual routine.

We should stay within our strength limit for a correct work out and do not force the execution every day for a secure muscle development. Working the outer part of the chest muscle, we need to have a larger grip on the barbell. This is usually easier and we can lift heavier weight. For working the inner side of the chest, the part of the muscles which are close to the sternum, we should have a close grip on the barbell. Here we have to be careful and stay with the elbows open far from the bench, to minimize the triceps inclusion. The barbell should be maintained above the chest muscles only. This way, you might have a slightly discomfort to your wrists when coming with the barbell too low. In general, during this execution, we cannot lower the barbell all the way to touch the chest. But, by pushing the barbell all way up above the chest, you should feel the inner part of the chest muscle working.

Bench press for triceps is a main exercise for the triceps muscles development. Laying down with the back on the bench, grab the barbell with both straight hands, bring it above the upper abdomen, bellow the chest muscles. Bring the barbell straight down vertically by bending the elbows. We must lower the elbows close to the body, even touching it and going lower than the laid upper body in both sides. It is very important not to keep the elbows open and not to go far of the body with them as in the case of a chest exercise. It is a must to be careful during the execution, to maintain the same straight path of the barbell when bringing it down and back up. You will have the feeling of slightly pushing the barbell further along with pushing upwards when lifting it. Do not forget the breathing is very important. Do not leave the air exhaled before you are back up with the barbell. You will not be able to place the barbell back on the rack, if you breath the air out too early.

At the arms work out, we might believe that first it is more important to start with biceps. Actually, the triceps is the first one who should be worked out. This is a bigger muscle and it might take more time and work to develop it. Once you succeeded making it big, the whole arm will look more powerful and strong. Triceps is made by 3 muscles and biceps is made by 2 muscles only.

Rows with a barbell (ramat) is another basic exercise working mostly the back. It has the ability to form the packs of muscles on your back. It builds up a powerful nice back. Doing rows, we are also working the biceps and the trapeze, but this is an exercise made for building the back muscles mainly.

We position ourselves with the legs apart one of the other and the knees bent. We grab the barbell in front of us with both hands, maintaining the back straight. When we start lifting it, we must pull the barbell with the back muscles first. The arms remain straight. The legs stay bent and still. The back is coming up only. When our upper body is half a way up, we help the back muscles with our arms to pull the barbell by bending the elbows. The bar is coming up touching the abdomen. We are continuing the rep by bringing down the upper body, using the back muscles first and then the arms. We stretch down the arms with the bar and execute the next consecutive rep. During the execution, we have to bring up the upper body till we are slightly higher than parallel to the ground. Do not lift the upper body higher than 75 degrees. When pulling the bar to the chest we are working the upper back mostly. When we bring the bar to the abdomen, we are working the lower half of the back mostly. The legs should stay in the same position for the whole exercise. Do not swing!

There is close grip to use when we are working the back muscles which are located close to the spine. We may also use large grip, when the outer dorsal is worked out the most. We should try both front barbell grip or back barbell grip as well. When using back barbell grip, the biceps is used during the exercise, too. When using front barbell grip, the trapezius and rear shoulder enter in the move as well.

Every time you work back muscles, you are also using your biceps anyway. Every time you work chest, you are also using your triceps. This is the reason that it is not recommended to work triceps in the same day with chest or biceps in the same day with back. We will not have enough strength to work out the second muscle group that is left at the end. We may even avoid this combination during 2 consecutive days. Now, if you take strong nutritional supplements, the rules will change because the muscle recovery would be much faster.

The descriptions above conclude the main exercises for muscle development. If you do these ones only, the success is guaranteed for gaining weight and strength. But, in order to have a complete work out and to involve more fibers, we need to do additional exercise.

There was an effective machine during the old times for doing rows. It had a T bar with an end where we could add discs and the weight we want. I did not see that machine in the modern gyms. We may improvise by using a regular barbell and adding discs at one of its ends.

There are lots of back exercises to do at the cable machines for the end of our workout when our strength is reduced. We should pull from all 3 angles towards us, from the upper side as well as from the front side and from the lower side. This way we have all the angles of the back muscles worked during the same work out. Do not forget, it does not matter what type of exercise you do, when you work the back muscles, in order to do a correct exercise, you have to start by pulling first with the back muscle and the arms should start bending afterwards. The arms are only used to have a complete exercise for the back. Our intention is not to build the arms right now. We could use the machines when we are not in a high mood for exercising or when we feel sick. The machines are for elderly or for the times when we experience a weak day.

In case we choose to use **dumbbells**, there are different types of working our back muscles with them. We could do rows in the same way as explained but using dumbbells this time. Or, we could lean upon a bench or anything else with one hand and the other hand would lift the dumbbell. The opposite knee may be placed on the bench for a better balance. We may do this exercise without leaning upon anything, having the knees bent and the upper body inclined forward. The leg from the same side with the arm that lifts the dumbbell, should be placed little backwards to maintain the balance. When coming up with the elbow, keep it close to the body. The arm and the elbow have to touch the upper body during this lifting. When going back down with the dumbbell, we must stretch the side dorsal very much. The arm should go down but forward in a straight line until the dumbbell is almost or even touching the ground. Do not execute a short stretch or do not use only the arm during the execution. By using the arm only, we are working the biceps mostly. Theoretically, the arm should serve as a moving hook for the purpose of developing the back dorsal. Think about cutting a tree trunk with a saw. This exercise should be executed exactly the same way. If we do not stretch enough the back, we will not work out the back muscle thoroughly. Unfortunately, this is a common mistake that many people do. Even some of the people who train for many years, they do the short stretch of their back. That is why some people go for years to the gym and they still look the same without seeing a progression. The back should permanently stay straight but not still and the buttock pushed out. In order to stretch the dorsal all the way down, try to go with the dumbbell as far as you can towards the floor but forward and do not drop it straight down. Lift the weight with your back muscle first while the arm is still straight in front of you. Only after you have pulled with the dorsal, you should use your arm and start bending it. Then, bring the elbow upwards, higher than the back.

In order to develop your back, you should try doing **pull ups** at the bar. Even if this is hard to do for a beginner, you should try it frequently. The body might get used to it and the new muscles will help you to succeed. We may try using forward grip on the bar. This will be harder to do. We may also try backward grip. This one involves more of the biceps usage and it should be used mostly for working out the biceps muscles. Using this grip, it is easier. When we do not stretch the arms all the way down, we are building the biceps only. If we want to work out the back muscles, too, the body should go down until we feel the dorsal stretching but do not relax in that position. We have to lift our body back up by pulling from the back muscles at first and then helping with our arms. We should do the lifting all the way up until the bar is in front of our face. The most effective for the back development is using the forward grip. When we are weaker, we could do this pull up exercise at the cable machine with the proper weight. If we are stronger and we feel we are able to lift a heavier weight than our body is, we may add another weight caught around the belt or between our feet during the pull up execution. We will need to add this additional weight, if only it is too easy for us to do correctly at least 10 pull ups per set.

Pushups are exercises where the chest and the triceps are used. We could do this as a warm up or at the end of your chest work out when you do not have much strength anymore. In case you are a beginner, this exercise should be one of your basic ones. If we keep our arms opened wide on the ground, we will work the outer sides of the chest. If we position the arms straight bellow the chest muscles, we will work the chest as a whole. When we place the arms closer to the upper body but bellow the lower side of the chest or upper abdomen, we are working the triceps mostly. Here we must bend our elbows backwards and not outwards as we do for working the chest.

A correct execution for pushups, involves the placement of our body in a straight line. We must face the ground, the buttock should be on the same straight line with our knees, spine and shoulders. Going down, we should not touch the ground and do not relax between the reps.

Deeps are exercises which work in a similar way. The difference is that they develop the lower side of the chest when we lean forward. They work out the triceps when our body stay straight vertically. During the execution we should lower our body until the arms are bent completely. Do not stop at half the way of the distance. Many people work deeps as a short move for different reasons. Unless you have no flexibility or this causes you joint pain, we do not have a reason to shorten the distance for the deeps execution. They were called deeps because they need to be executed deep.

Backward arms extensions for triceps using the barbell. We may work out with a straight bar or a W bar. The muscles work in slightly different angles. It is helpful to switch between these choices time to time. The exercise starts with the bar grabbed by the both straight arms above the head. The elbows have to touch the ears or be close to them. They must stay still during the whole execution. Meanwhile, both forearms are moving the bar up and down. We lower the bar behind the head until the forearms touch the biceps. Do not relax or rest anytime during the set! During the up and down move, do not open the elbows! We may have that tendency when lifting the weight behind the head. Keep the elbows close to the ears all the time! If you are not able to lift the weight without keeping the elbows in a correct way, decrease the weight used. It is too heavy for you right now.

This exercise may be done from standing or sitting position. It may be done from laying down, as well. We need to warm up good before this exercise. It is a little bit risky when doing it uncontrolled. It happened when certain people have been already warmed up but the injury occurred anyway and a tendon broke. It is recommended that this exercise to be done with a lower weight in order to have it better under control.
Also, when we work triceps to the cable machine, the forearms should be moved all way up until they touch the biceps and all way down till the arms are completely straight. The elbows stay still for the whole execution.

Flies (fluturi) for chest is an exercise which works the chest muscle in its width. We use dumbbells laying on a bench. The bench may be lift at an oblique angle or straight horizontally. Facing upward with the dumbbells in the hands, we need to have the elbows slightly bent. Lower the arms in both sides on a semicircle path. The arms should stay curved for the whole set, the way they were placed initially. As we bring the arms down at the sides, the outer chest is working more when we let the arms lower than the level of the bench.

For developing the inner chest, the part of the muscle which is located near the sternum, we should have the dumbbells touching each other when lifting the arms above the body. There is another exercise in the same position, but instead of doing the semicircle movement, we need to push the dumbbells on a straight line above the chest. Bringing the arms straight up with the dumbbells close one to the other, try using the inner part of the chest muscle more than the arms. Being a female, it would be helpful not to get the arms too low in the sides. It might cause the development of both breasts too far one of the other. Some females have this problem without doing any chest exercise. By working the inner part of the chest muscle, we could help correcting this issue.

Shoulder press is one of the main exercises we could do for shoulder development. The execution is made from sitting or standing. The safest way for our back is working out sitting, on a bench which has a back support with an additional rack for the barbell at the back top. The rack is helpful for an easier pick up and placing back the barbell before and after the set. Even if the barbell may be picked and brought up without the help of a rack, the rack would help when using heavier weights. When doing the best trial with our maximum strength and working without a partner, that rack is a must. Anyway, after you manage to bring the barbell above the head and keep it with your hands straight, lower the barbell in a straight line down till it is at the level of the ears. When bringing it in the front of your head, the front side of your shoulders is mostly working. We should do the exercise by lowering the barbell in both sides: front and back. The workout for the front shoulders, should be followed by a workout for the back shoulders during the next shoulder day. It depends which side of the shoulders you may think it needs more work done, you may insist on that side.

Shoulder flies is an exercise where our goal is to develop the rear side of the shoulder or the width of it. Leaning forward with the upper body straight, the legs should stay bent. Keep shoulders and the buttock backwards for a correct position with not accidents. Lift the dumbbells with both hands forming a semicircle path along both sides. The elbows should stay slightly bent for the whole execution. When the arms are up in both sides, bring the elbows little higher than the shoulders level. Do not swing the upper body! If we move the upper body during the execution, we will need to reduce the dumbbells' weight. It is too heavy for us! Like any exercise where we need to lean forward the upper body, we have to keep the back straight and not hunched. I noticed many beginners do this mistake. I have goose bumps on my skin when I see them. It is a must to avoid damaging the back. The spine has a very important role within our structure.

For an easier set up, we may lean our chest and stomach upon an oblique bench and try to lift the elbows backwards in that semicircle, higher than the level of the bench.
We may also work the rear shoulders, one at a time by laying on a side on a horizontal bench. We are using the arm on top only. It has to lift the dumbbell with the elbow slightly bent.

Shoulder flies from a complete vertically position will work the shoulders in their width. The position of the legs will be the same as described for the rear shoulder flies. But, the upper body should stay straight up for now. The arms need to be lift in both sides higher than the level of the shoulders. The elbows stay slightly bent. When they got to be high up, they need to stay turned upwards. The wrists should stay soft and the hands dropped down. The position of the arms should be the same way as when you pour water out of a glass with your hands, having your arms up on the sides. This way we make sure we are using mostly our shoulders and not the arms as much, when we execute the move. When we are working a certain muscle, we should stay with our mind thinking of that muscle, to feel that one is working. We do not want to believe we are working one muscle but actually the muscle that is really working is a different one. This should apply for every exercise we do. In order to grow the muscular mass for each group of muscles separately and at its highest effectiveness, we need to focus at what we work on, mentally and physically at the time of the execution.

We may lift the dumbbells in front of us with the arms straight and the elbows slightly bent. This is an exercise for the front side of the shoulders. When coming up with the dumbbells, they should be lift higher than the level of our shoulders or at least at the level of the shoulders. The arms should be lift alternatively, one at a time. For a better balance and a correct posture, the knees should stay little bent with 10 cm distance between them.

Leg press is a machine that everybody knows it. It is probably not necessary to explain how to use it. But, there are few things that I could mention here. The machine may be built to work the legs from different angles. The angle of a leg press determines the level of heaviness for that machine and implicitly the weight you are able to use when working out with it. Does not matter the angle of the machine when we choose the spot for placing our feet on it to push. We may place the feet on the upper or the lower side. By placing them lower, we are working more the quadriceps, the pressure is more on the lower quads. Placing them higher, we are working more the rear upper legs, the hamstrings and some glutes. It is understandable we cannot relax between the reps. For having a continuous move, we may not straighten the legs all the way to get the knees locked. As any other exercise, the moves should flow controlled one after another.

Lunges (fandari) are very important for our legs development. They should be included among the basic exercises. We may do them using the barbell on top of the shoulders or using the dumbbells. The upper body should stay straight when walking. The distance between the steps should be as large as we are able to do a step. Do not rest and stand between the steps! The movement should be continuous as a giant would naturally have his step after step.

Lounges may also be executed in place with just one step forward and back, followed by the other leg with a step forward and back. The execution may be done with one leg for a few reps, followed by the other leg with its reps. Lounges that are done in place are not so effective as the ones done walking with huge steps. When we do the large steps consequently, we pull harder from the glutes, quads and hamstrings. If we are not use to do them or we increase the weight for that specific workout, we will surely have muscular fever the second day at the latest. This is a sign of an effective legs workout.

Biceps curls and leg extensions (flexii/extensii) are good to be done at the end of the workout in order to have a thorough legs session. I do not need to describe these exercises as they are worked on the machines. But, I had to mention them because they have their specific role during the workout. They have an importance when we are trying to get more ripped by exercising to them with more reps per set. This is especially before a competition.

Calves should not be anytime avoided out of our legs workout. There are couple of machines that work calves. For example, the one which works the calves from sitting position and the one from standing. I prefer the machine from standing but unfortunately, I have not seen it in all the gyms. This is the reason I had to improvise different ways of working calves. Especially when you compete, this group of muscles would impress the judges, too.

Abdominal muscles should be worked from different angles. This is considered a small group of muscles, even if it involves lots of muscles coming from different angles. We should treat the stomach muscles as we treat any important group of muscles on our body. We need to work the upper abdomen, the lower abs and the obliques. Usually, for crunches we need to do a short move in order to form the abs thick and protruding. We do not want the abdominal muscles to be long on top of a protruding tummy. In order to work the lower abs, we may stay hung of a bar and lift the legs. We could bend the knees during the execution or lift them straight. For working the obliques, we should lift our bent legs in a side and in the other. The same way, we may exercise on a straight bench bringing both up, the upper body and the legs in the same time. When doing crunches hung or on the bench, we need to learn to keep our balance. This is the hardest part for the beginners. Once this become easier, you may try adding some weight like a dumbbell between your feet. There are different machines with cables that you can alternate at a couple of months. A simple but lucrative exercise is even the one where you are working the abs on the floor. The idea is, where ever you work out, the movement must be short. Do not forget to breath correctly at each move. Usually we exhale when the upper body and the legs come close together and inhale when these both are apart.

In order to develop the muscles more, we should change the type of the exercise once per 2 months. When we want to develop our strength for an exercise, it is good to do it at many consecutive workouts for that specific group of muscles. But, when an individual has the same salary every year with no incentive or bonus, his struggle for developing his qualities gets capped. The same way it happens when our muscles get used to one type of exercise or to the same weight used, they stop growing. This is a natural thing that occurs for everything.

When having the feet hooked up on a railing or on some handles and the rest of the body is hanging upside down vertically or on an oblique bench, we may work the upper stomach muscles the most. To be more effective, we should place the hands behind the head. We may use a weight to make it harder and develop thicker abs. Usually, the upper abs are the ones who develop first anyway. Mostly, we have to insist on the lower abs. Many beginners say: "I do not want to develop a think abdomen". Do not be afraid. We are talking now about muscle development and not about fat development. Remember, if you have more muscle mass, you will be able to lose fat easier.

Triceps and biceps are smaller group of muscles. They

are worked and developed anyway when exercising the back, chest or shoulders. But when we wish to compete, we have to work them as well, to form them separately and finish their shape with real cuts. I mentioned earlier about the basic exercises for triceps. There exist isolation exercises as well, which have their role in the development, especially when we want to define the muscles that are already there. An isolation exercise for triceps starts by leaning forward with the upper body and the legs bent. We are trying to lift a dumbbell with one arm near the upper body. Keep your elbow fixed and close to the upper body. Lift the dumbbell backwards with the forearm only to make a straight arm. Then, the forearm comes down until is touching the biceps. During the execution, only the forearm is moving back and forth. The rest of the body should stay still for the whole set.

We may work the biceps using the straight bar, W bar or with dumbbells from standing or sitting. When you work out standing, the knees should be bent and the upper body slightly leaning forward for a better balance. The elbows should stay fixed all the time near the upper body. The forearms are moving only, up and down. Do not swing! Do not move the elbows back and forth! When working from the sitting position, the elbows should stay fixed against the quad. If using the bench with a support for the arm, do not lift the arm in the air or swing the body. Doing that, we are showing our incompetency for lifting that heavy weight. We should change it to an easier one. When we are working a certain muscle, we have to make sure we are working out that specific muscle only.

There are couple of exercises that many people, especially females do in the gym, that are not recommended to be done. They develop an ugly body shape when done frequently. One of them is bending the upper body in a side with a dumbbell in the hand. Legs straight and still. When finishing the reps for that side, the dumbbell needs to be switched to the other hand for bending the upper body in the other side. This exercise builds muscles around the waist, especially in the sides above the hips. We do not want that. The waist needs to be thin. In that area, the muscles will develop anyway by doing exercises for the other groups of muscles. Moreover, if we have a lot of muscles built up on the sides of the waist, we need to keep a layer of minimum fat, minimum water and toxins to cover it forever. Otherwise it will be terrible. All of us know how hard is for the majority of us to keep the fat layer low on top of our waist all the time. Having a thin waist, we are not forced to build very wide shoulders. The V shape of our upper body will still be there.

These are all the exercises that we need for a complete muscle development and strength. There are many other exercises using machines or cables that I have not described. Those ones, I am sure, you will figure them out by yourselves. If not, we could take a certain trainer to help with changing the pin at the weight machine for us and pay him for his hard work.

Additionally, I saw and tried few years ago some examples of new generation machines. They even work on our behalf! We do not have to strain almost at all when exercise with them. Indeed, they take a lot of pressure out of our joints when we use them. But, they take a lot of pressure out of the weight, too. They are good for the age of 85+, when the joints are very brittle. I do not want to give the name of the brand and do a bad advertisement. Unfortunately, this is what the modern world has started to offer us. If you choose using machines for a real muscle development, I would recommend using the oldest and rusty ones. You are lucky if you still find them. I personally had the chance to try some very old machines at a poor gym in my country. They were little different than the usual machines we use at a regular gym. They were working the muscles almost like the free weights. When adding a little bit of weight on them, it was much heavier to lift as at a regular machine. That gym should be called "Rusty but the Gym of Real Gold".

Chapter 7

Nutritional Supplements

In order to gain muscles or to lose fat we may help ourselves by using nutritional supplements. These additional foods may also be used in case we are sick and we cannot ingest enough nutrients for our body to perform his tasks correctly. Or, for the simple fact that we need more protein to gain muscle mass. We need proteins, carbohydrates and fats to have a strong and long life. But, when we eat enough protein as regular food, too many bad fats are coming together with it. We cannot eat a piece of meat containing protein only. Even if it is a lean meat, it still has fat, too. Fats are also good but we need to limit them. To have under control the amount of fat, carbs or protein that we introduce in our body, we have to eat both regular food and nutritional supplements. We must exercise as well, at least 3 or 4 times per week for about 30 to 45 minutes. All these are related when talking about staying fit but healthy.

There are nutritional supplements that help us having the necessary protein intake per day. Others are helping our body to have the necessary amount of good fat. There are supplements which help reduce the adipose layer or to increase our muscular mass. This chapter will list all the different types of them. The chapter will not comprehend medicines or pills that should be taken by prescription from the doctor. I will resume to natural supplements that everybody may find at the natural products stores. Some countries have them at the regular supermarkets and nutritional supplements shops including their online websites.

Losing weight supplements

L-Carnitine is an amino acid who helps reducing the adipose layer. It usually needs to be taken 15 minutes before the aerobic exercise as running, biking, swimming, jump rope and other. When you take it before exercise, you will sweat more during the cardio session and you will have more energy to fulfill the session. By using it, the body starts using energy from the fat much more and earlier during the exercise. For example, when running, we are feeling more energized and we start losing fat after 5 or 10 minutes of running. Without the use of L-Carnitine, we start to lose fat after 15 minutes only, after the time we have already got rid of the glycogen from the muscles. This supplement has an important role for losing the fat, as it helps to transport the bad fat acids to the cellular mitochondria where it produces energy. This only happens when L-Carnitine is consumed together with doing physical exercise.

Our body produces by itself this amino acid but in small quantities or we may take it from certain foods we eat as the red meat or the milk. It helps the hepatic function. But otherwise, as any other food or supplement used in excess, this one has its side effects when taken more than 4 grams per day. Usually we should take about 500 mg to 1000 mg for 1 time or 2 times per day, the times we do the aerobic in order to lose less muscles. We may take it before the weight lifting workout as we wish. This amino acid is used mostly for the purpose of losing fat, but it also helps in a certain proportion for the muscle mass.

Acetyl-L-Carnitine is a derivative of L-Carnitine. Its action seems to be quicker in the system than L- ·

Carnitine. Besides of its benefit related to losing fat, this is recommended for a healthy heart and brain. It helps with the memory function, too. The doses are the same as for L-Carnitine.

Omega 3 may be found by itself or in a specific combination with Omega 6 and Omega 9. This is a recommended supplement for losing fat. It reduces the bad cholesterol from the blood vessels. By cleaning the body, it helps to get rid of the adipose layer as well. Taking 2000 mg of these good fats per day and especially before a fatty meal, they do not allow our system to store new fat cells from the food we eat. It is not advisable to use more than 3000 mg Omega in total. It increases the risk for bleeding. We can find the supplement in fish oils, flex oils, nuts or others.

Inulin is a polysaccharide which helps the digestion by its fiber content. It slows down the intestine absorption of the bad nutrients and increases the absorption of the minerals as calcium and magnesium. The inulin has vegetable origins and acts like the prebiotics inside the intestines. That means, it does not digest in the small intestine and goes down in the large intestine where ferments, forming the good bacteria. It maintains a good intestinal flora. This fiber has the ability to reduce the food appetite. It cleans the liver of toxins, increasing the immunity. After consuming inulin, the blood sugar level remains unmodified. We may find it as a powder form. It tastes neuter, slightly sweet, less sweet than sugar. It is a good choice to sweeten our coffee with it, the tea or adding to the food. We may use 5 grams, 3 times per day.

Green tea works as an energizer because it contains the theine which gets spread in the blood for a period of 6 to 8 hours. Its effect is not so strong as drinking a coffee, but it is longer. The coffee releases its caffeine effect for 2 to 3 hours only. The green tea reduces the damage made by the free radicals. Used along with other different products, green tea helps for losing weight as well.

Choline is one of the B vitamins which activates the responsible hormones to consume fats. It also helps the liver to dispose the unwanted fats. This vitamin is effective for the brain function and the age-related memory problems. Usually we may find it in combination with other losing weight substances or in products containing other B vitamins as inositol. As any other supplement or food, the usage of too much choline may give bad side effects, as well. Our body produces choline by itself, but it might not be enough as a nutrient for our system, especially when lots of hard workouts are included in our daily activities. We could find natural choline in foods like beef, chicken livers, peanuts and others. We need enough choline to be able to produce methionine.

Methionine is an amino acid who has an important role for fat disintegration. The adrenaline hormone can be produced in the methionine presence only. The adrenaline transports and eliminates a high amount of the adipose layer existing on the top of our tummies. We may take methionine naturally from fish, chicken and yogurts.

Linoleic acid is a fat acid (Omega 6) which cannot be produced by our system. But, his existence is important for our intestines because it dries the intestines lining who retains fat during the digestion process. This way, less fats enter into the blood circulation and the hormones that have a role as fat consumers, reach faster the adipose cells. Linoleic acid is found in flex seeds and sunflower seeds (oil). We may find it in different nutritional supplements products, as well.

CLA stands for Conjugated Linoleic Acid. This is the Omega 6 with double bonds to the fatty acid molecule. This polyunsaturated fatty acid is very healthy for us but we can take it from the outside of the body only. It exists mostly in beef and dairy.

Researchers found it helpful for its anticancer properties. CLA is a strong antioxidative and anticatabolic. It is a good stimulator for the immune system. But, when taken above the recommended dose, it may cause indigestion.

This is often used during the fat loss diets because it maintains a high metabolic rate but it also protects the muscle mass, having the ability to increase it. CLA has a benefic impact for decreasing the bad cholesterol and the triglycerides and reduces the risk of having food allergy.

A lack of CLA may cause a pronounced fattening. It is impossible to take all the necessary CLA from the regular food. We would need to ingest a way too big quantity of food for that. In order to have 5 grams of CLA per day, we should consume an amount of food that comes with additionally 500 grams of saturated fat together, which is way too much for our body. The only way of ingesting pure CLA without additional bad fats is to use CLA supplements.

Vitamin C seems to help for the losing fat process along with the other benefits it offers.

Taurine is an amino acid who has many benefits within our system. Along with other tasks, it is responsible to

release the hormones who help to the fat transportation. We may find taurine in fish, shrimp or see food. This amino acid regulates the digestion functions and the cholesterol levels by forming the gall bladder's salts. It also enhances the cardiac functions for those who are predisposed to an irregular heart rate. This amino acid has to exist in a large quantity inside the heart muscle for a good functioning. Taurine helps those who have frequent muscular cramps by bringing the minerals and electrolytes to the muscle tissue.
Taurine plays also a small role as an energizer but the energy drinks producers usually use different compounds to form taurine. They do not extract it straight from the natural sources. An energy drink has a high effect mostly because of its caffeine content, rather than its taurine inclusion.

All these supplements with a role in losing the fat are effective only when we exercise regularly!

Gaining weight supplements

Protein powder may contain different quantities of protein and carbohydrates. In order to gain muscle mass, we should use a powder containing at least 40% - 50% protein, because protein is the base for the muscles to grow. We need carbs, too for their benefits in terms of the energy supply. There are supplements containing **whey**, which is a protein with quick absorption. It may be taken anytime during the day on empty stomach. It is important to avoid taking it in the same time with other amino acids or protein coming from the regular food. A product is made in such a way, for our body to be able to absorb it fully. The producer chooses a good match for the quantities of each amino acid in the protein powder to have a perfect assimilation. When we do use another supplement or food with it, in the same 10 minutes interval, the quantities of certain amino acids will change and they will not form the complete protein anymore. Our system will not be able to assimilate it and we may lose a big amount of those nutrients. The body will just get rid of it, out of the system through the intestines passage. When a lonely amino acid enters in our body and wants to become part of a protein, it travels around to look for its match in order to form the complete protein. He is worried if he will not find his perfect partners, he will have to leave that system. This is the reason for the manufactories to pick the right amino quantities and offer on the market the proper amino acids formula inside their products.

There is protein powder that contains casein. This is still a milk product as well as the whey is. The difference is that the **casein** has a slow absorption. It is recommended to be taken in the evening. During the night, we do not eat anything for many hours. We do not want our muscles to enter in catabolism. The casein will feed them gradually throughout the night.

On the market you may find products containing only **amino acids** under the form of pills, powder or liquid. The liquid is easier to assimilate. Amino acids are usually easy to assimilate by our system because they are already the broken form of the proteins. They are the compounds of the proteins. They may be made from milk, beef or soy. You may take amino acids anytime during the day on empty stomach and take them about 10 or 15 minutes apart of the other foods or supplements. We may take them once or two times per night for catabolism prevention when we have a strenuous physical activity during the day and we want to gain muscle mass or for a bodybuilder. There are different brands on the market. We should choose the one that has a higher dose of each amino acid. We should always read the labels even if it may take more time to spend in the store. There are certain amino acids manufactured separately, because of their strong effects when taken in a big quantity and apart of the other amino acids.

BCAA is a product that contains the main essential amino acids: leucine, isoleucine and valine. These amino acids cannot be produced by our body but they are necessary to exist in the system. We have to take them from the food or supplements. These branched chain amino acids are some of the main building blocks for our muscles. They help to recover the muscles after an intense workout. We find Leucine in a higher proportion than the other 2 amino acids in BCAA. We may also find Leucine by itself as a separate product to buy. We have to take this amino acid on empty stomach as well, in order to be assimilated well in the body.

HMB is another product which is related to Leucine. It is a Leucine metabolite. When our body breaks down Leucine, we are using HMB. It is an anticatabolic supplement. We may take it from fish and grapefruit or as a nutritional supplement from the store.

Creatine is naturally produced inside our body from other amino acids. But, we may also take it from food as the red meat. We may find it as phosphate creatine or monohydrate creatine. The phosphate creatine may give a reaction of the skin as pins and needles or redness. I personally did not like to use any types of creatine for multiple reasons. It gives you strength but it also retains a lot of water between muscles and skin. It is not recommended to be used before competitions because may inhibits the body ability to become ripped. During the off season, we may use creatine for its benefits. For a better absorption, it is recommended to be taken together with something sweet as dextrose or fructose. Creatine gives energy to the cells in the muscle tissue. ATP (adenosine triphosphate) is the engine for the muscles functioning. For a muscle to contract, the ATP molecule must give him the energy by breaking her chains. When the muscle cell finishes her ATP, it is not able to contract herself anymore into an environment with no oxygen. The heavy lifting workout is done into an anaerobic environment. Here comes the role of the creatine phosphate in our system.

Muscles use glycogen during the anaerobic workout when lifting heavy weights. Studies have been showing that Creatine helps to stock the glycogen into the muscle and prevent muscle atrophy.

Many people speak about the need of a loading phase with Creatine at the beginning and then a maintenance phase. I personally do not think this has an importance. We may take Creatine 5 grams at a time, before exercise without any initial loading.

L-Glutamine is known as a strong supplement when taken separately. It is the most abundant amino acid in the muscle. Glutamine is 60% of the amino acids in the muscle content. It is advisable to be taken 5 to 10 mg before our workout to gives us energy and the same amount after workout to replenish the lost energy, the glycogen from the muscles. Glutamine is not an essential amino acid because our system is able to synthesize it in high quantities from other amino acids (from branched chain amino acids). During the stress conditions, our body is not able to synthesize it in sufficient quantities. That is why, we should take it from outside as a nutritional supplement.

L-Glutamine has multiple roles in our system. It is a donor of nitrogen during the glucosamine sulfate synthesis for joints nourishing. It is a liver protector. It helps to break down the proteins at the kidney level by maintaining the acids balance. It facilitates the release of a small quantity of the growth hormones. It is a major source of fuel for the immune system cells. It sustains the cellular hydration, favoring the cell's anabolic activity. It helps to the glucose release during the workouts preventing the hypoglycemia. These are only few of the many reasons we should take glutamine. When we get stressed out, the hormone called cortisol appears. L-Glutamine blocks the cortisol activity inside the muscles.

L-Arginine is an amino acid with an important role in the protein synthesis. It is needed for the development of all the body tissues. It helps the liver. Without an enough quantity in our system, the occurrence of muscle development and fat loss is difficult. L-Arginine intensifies the growth hormone release. This amino acid generates the nitric oxide in our body which is very important for blood vessels dilatation and relaxation. When building our body nicely, we want to have tonus in the muscles and be pumped up. Arginine offers you this effect. Moreover, it gives you a lot more strength during the workout and you will see more protruding veins on the body for the time when you are exercising. This is also an important quality we need to have during a competition.

Arginine is not an essential amino acid. Our body can produce it by itself or we can take it from eggs, meat and other proteins. Taking Arginine as supplement is very helpful. We may take 1000 mg before going to the gym and we will see a big difference for the quality of our workout.

This amino acid has many benefits, but also side effects when taken over the recommended dose. L-Arginine helps to get rid of the ammoniac which is a debris for our system. It also helps during the treatment for patients having cardiac insufficiency. It is good to ask the opinion of a medical professional if your health is not perfectly fine before use. You may find it in the store under the form of pills, powder or liquid.

L-Citrulline malate is an amino acid who raises the Arginine quantity in the blood, which produces more nitric oxide. When is more nitric oxide, it brings more blood to the muscle tissue during the physical exercise. This allows them to resist much more under pressure. Muscles will be more pumped up during the heavy lifting. The component called malate, combats the physical tiredness, transforming the lactic acid into energy. Malate helps us get rid of the muscular fever. Citrulline malate also gives a stronger immune system against respiratory infections when an athlete may become weak because of physical exhaustion. We may find this amino acid into a formula together with other amino acids or by himself.

L-Carnitine is the amino acid who not only helps for losing weight but it is good to be used by those who gain hard their muscles. L-Carnitine gives energy and more strength. More strength helps us working with heavier weights, fact that fructifies in more muscular mass. A bigger muscular mass means a higher metabolic rate which facilitates fat burning. Muscular mass is in a relationship with losing fat. That is why I had to mention here about the both processes. To conclude, L-Carnitine helps to recover easier after the hard workouts.

Along with the benefits that I have mentioned at the section Lose Weight Products, this amino acid also decreases the problems of the bone mass aging related and it is helpful for male fertility by increasing the sperm count. It also stands against allergies and cold symptoms by preventing the cell degradation in the presence of the free radicals.

Royal Jelly is the milky of the Queen Bee. It may be found by itself or together with other supplements as **pollen, propolis, ginseng**. All these are energizers and help for the immune system, but they have numerous other qualities as well, which I do not list here. It is known that they help fight against cancer and they are a huge support for muscle mass growth. In the past, when there were not nutritional supplements products as we benefit today of, athletes had built muscles by using bee products and powder milk. Royal Jelly contains amino acids with unique structure which are rarely met into other natural foods. It was discovered that Royal Jelly also contains some testosterone as well as progesterone that helps with masculine and feminine fertility, but also with gaining strength when lifting weights and resistance when running.

ZMA stands for zinc, magnesium and vitamin B6. This supplement contains higher quantities of zinc. When an athlete does strenuous workouts, his muscles deplete quick of these minerals. Without enough magnesium and vitamin B6, we may do muscular cramps or we may not be able to respond easy to the stress situations. A lack of magnesium may negatively affect the testosterone production. Usually, ZMA contains 450 mg of magnesium, which is a good amount for people who have hard workouts. On the other hand, zinc is an important mineral involved into many hormones activity as insulin, growth hormone, testosterone or estrogen. Studies have shown that, those who train hard are predisposed to zinc deficits. ZMA contains 30 mg of zinc. Vitamin B6 may reduce the cortisol, the stress hormone, fact that could benefit the testosterone level.

Whether we are men or women, we have certain amount of estrogen and an amount of testosterone. Both, women and men we want to increase the testosterone level when building muscle mass. But, if we already have these minerals from ZMA at a high amount in our body, this product will probably not help. We may still consume it for the other health benefits it offers.

Beta-alanine is not an essential but an important amino acid for the body. When it meets histidine, it forms carnosine. Our muscles need carnosine for their strength and resistance. The muscular fiber has the ability to contract herself for a longer period of time when we have more carnosine inside it. Beta-alanine offers both benefits: increases the muscle mass and decreases the adipose layer. There are studies that affirm, when this amino acid is combined with creatine, it may have a

better effect strength wise. We may use 1 or 2 grams of beta-alanine or carnosine before the workout or/and after it. We may take till 6 grams per day. Carnosine helps stabilize the muscle PH by reducing the acidity inside it. When the PH drops below the alkaline limit, the muscular performance drops, too.
We do not have to take histidine supplements along with it. Our muscles should already have enough histidine formed. If you are not a vegetarian, you should have the histidine quantity that is necessary for the muscle to form carnosine. Taking simple beta-alanine is the best choice because when we take carnosine, our body will transform it anyway in beta-alanine and later on, it forms carnosine. The performance benefits may increase in 2 or 3 weeks as we supplement our muscles with it or we may see a difference after the first day we take. Everybody functions different. Carnosine is a precursor of the nitric oxide. That is why we should see a vasodilation during our workout for the time period we use beta-alanine.

Beta-ecdysterone is a substance which protects the plants against insects. People use it for its anabolic qualities. It needs to be taken in high quantities to feel an effect for the muscle growth, but the supplements that are manufactured, contain a perfect dose that works with human body. It does not classify as a hormone. It mostly helps with protein synthesis for muscle growth. It also stimulates the fat loss and our metabolism. The recommended dose is between 200 mg to 500 mg.

There are some other supplements that raise naturally the testosterone level and contain strong substances. **D-aspartic acid** is an amino acid found in neuroendocrine tissue. It helps the testicles to produce more testosterone. This way, males are able to build more muscle mass and lose fat easier.

Tribulus Terrestris is another supplement for raising the testosterone level. It is extracted from a plant. There exist many other supplements that can increase the testosterone level and for sure new ones will appear on the market. Only by trying them, we can see which one works for our body. Stay between the instructed doses!

We do not have to take all these products every day. We should take some for a while and then change to others. It will be good and more effective for our body to be shocked by the changes. Otherwise, the system will be over solicited with breaking down so many products, when too many supplements are taken. It is possible that our body will not answer the way we want when being overwhelmed. We should use no more than the recommended doses. Read the labels!

Other useful supplements:

MSM (methyl-sulfonyl-methane) is a supplement that helps a lot with the joints pain. A certain quantity of Sulphur, brought to our system together with Calcium, does miracles to our joints. Sulphur is a component of the Glutathione which is a protein who acts as the most important antioxidants that our body produces. Additionally, Glutathione is the main detoxifier of the liver. Taking MSM will help the liver as well as it recovers our cartilage getting rid of the inflammation that occurred around it. Do not stop exercising! When the joints are moving, MSM is brought to the area and adds the nutrient to the cartilage. We need to be consistent and take it every day for 3 months. The 3 following months are necessary for a break. We will start again to take another 3 months of MSM after the break. In about 2 years of keep doing that cycle, the cartilage should heal if we have been also exercising but no more than the discomfort limit. It depends how severe is the problem and how much of the cartilage is destroyed. The dose should be 2000 mg per day. There are certain supplements containing small doses. They do not have the ability to heal. Moreover, a cartilage health problem needs a long time before it may be resolved completely. If we take a 3 months period of this treatment only, we will not have a complete healing. MSM works very good together with glucosamine, chondroitin, Boswellia Serrata and collagen extract or shark cartilage. It is recommended to be taken a supplement complex that contains also other components along with MSM for a maximum effect. I personally believe, MSM is the most powerful of all the products for joints recovery.

There are studies about **Glucosamine** that it replenishes the nutrients in the cartilage, forming back the part that got destroyed. By having a poor nutrition or by exercising and running a lot, the cartilage in the joints may degrade and the synovial liquid may be reduced. Glucosamine has the quality of forming this liquid for a better lubrication during the movements. This substance is natural when extracted from the conch shells. Binding a water molecule, we sustain the humidity and the density of the synovial liquid. That will maintain the lubrication inside the joint. During the different movements we do, this liquid gets into and out of the cartilage that wraps the end of the bone. The liquid fills the cartilage with nutrients and it helps with releasing out of it all the formed residues. That is why we need to do physical exercise during the time we take glucosamine and chondroitin.

When the joints are cracking doing noise, they release the air caught in between the cartilages and they line themselves. That is not a bad thing. When this noise is present together with swelling, pain or redness, here is an issue that needs to be treated.

If we do not take measures at the first signs of pain, the joints will degrade much more and the muscles around the joints will get weaker.

Chondroitin is extracted from the shark or bovine cartilage. It helps the human cartilage to retain water and it may reverse the cartilage loss. It is recommended to be used together with glucosamine and other joint helpers.

Our blood transports the nutrients to the cells. The cartilage is not irrigated with blood. The blood's role is replaced by the water. In this case, the water brings the nutrients to the cartilage. When our joints get worn out, the sulphate chondroitin in the cartilage decreases, the joint aptitude to retain water decreases and it reduces the tissues elasticity. Here comes the need for using the nutritional supplement.

Collagen is an important protein in our body which is needed by our cartilages, bones, ligaments, tendons and skin. We may find it at any store. The recommended dose is written on the pack or ask a pharmacist.

Hyaluronic Acid stimulates the collagen synthesis and it retains water, helping to hydration. This acid is used for cosmetic purposes, too.

L-Cysteine is an amino acid that it is also good for our skin. It contributes to the skin elasticity because it helps to the collagen production and it repairs the hair and nails. We often find this supplement together with Glutamine, Methionine and Taurine for a strong immune system sustaining the athletes muscular mass. L-Cysteine offers benefits related to detox. It contains Sulphur and it is a component of the glutathione. It protects our body against the free radicals and it is good for releasing the mucus out of the breathing system.

When we are stressed out, the body produces more cortisol. Sometimes we are not able to keep the cortisol under control and this may affect our shape, decrease our muscle mass and increase the adipose layer. It may contribute to water and toxins retention under the skin and we get covered. Especially when we prepare for a competition or we are on the stage, we want the least water retention in between the muscle and skin. We have to get rid of the stress. There are natural supplements who help us towards this matter.

5-HTP (5-hydroxytryptophan) is recommended for the maintenance of our nervous system health. It increases the brain serotonin levels for bringing the desire and communication capacity of an individual who lost his interest in doing things. It induces the calm and self-confidence. It brings relaxation and helps with the sleeping problems. It reduces the number of waking ups during the night by raising the melatonin levels. It reduces the excess of carbs consumption caused by the emotional disturbances. 5-HTP is a naturally occurring substance derived from the seeds of Griffonia Simplicifolia, a West African medicinal plant. Many times, the factories that produce it, do not use naturally extracted substances. They chemically manufacture them in the labs.

GABA (gamma-aminobutyric acid) is another supplement which helps with relaxation and sleeping. It is an amino acid that functions as a neurotransmitter in the brain and supports brain function. It induces a calm mood and supports the function of the pituitary gland which facilitates a restful sleep. In addition, GABA has been shown to stimulate a 400% increase in human growth hormone production. It helps recover after exercise and effort.

Melatonin is one of the best substances produced by our body which induces restful sleep. We need more melatonin present in the body during evening when it is the time to fall asleep. Sometimes, this strong antioxidant is not produced enough by our system at the right time. Here comes helpful to add the nutritional supplement. Moreover, this supplement decreases the bad cholesterol in the body, promoting health for our heart. It reinforces our immune system and it delays the aging process. The melatonin level may start to diminish by the time we are teenagers. Melatonin is also safe in small doses for children but should not be used before asking a medical professional. In US we may find it in the pills form in regular supermarkets with a dose of 1 mg melatonin/day for infants.

Moreover, the melatonin production in our system happens when we are in a dark environment only. It is inhibited even at dust, at the edge of the day. Researchers have demonstrated that checking our e-mails before going to bed, it has the same effect as drinking a coffee.

There are other supplements good for us on the market but the ones above are the basic to build a healthy and looking good body shape. The protein and simple amino acids should be taken on empty stomach at all times for a complete absorption. Follow the instructions and doses on the packs. Usually if one takes more than the recommended dose, it will not be more useful. The body will eliminate the quantity he does not need at that moment or this might even affect the system in a wrong way. We do not want to waste these supplements because they are not cheap but very helpful. On another hand, people who have a larger muscle mass volume or they are taller, they need to use a larger quantity of proteins or amino acids for muscle growth. But, everything that you take have to be good controlled. When you get confused ask a health care professional about the doses you need. Moreover, some of us might be allergic to different substances, be lactose intolerant or get sick because of certain compounds a product may contain. The recommended doses are meant to be used by a healthy individual who exercise regularly, where the body responds exactly like in theory and after the usual standards.

Chapter 8

Risks and Benefits in the Civilized World

Nowadays it is very hard to avoid the use of chemicals and growth hormones and to take the proper nutrition from the regular food. Chemicals are everywhere, in the fruits and vegetables, in the meats, in the air we breathe in the buildings because of the conditioned air system, pollution outside the buildings and others I will mention in this chapter. Chemicals form toxins in our body which is a reason of the illnesses. Toxins make harder the losing fat process. Modern world, modern cellulite... The layer of fat that has that look of the orange skin is formed from toxins, water and fat. If the toxins did not exist, the water and fat would disappear much easier. When there are toxins, the process of losing that unwanted layer is slower. In order to avoid having toxins in the body, we have to avoid using chemicals. As I mentioned, these days it is very hard to avoid chemicals. This is a dangerous reason for more and more people to be predisposed for gaining fat. If they do not take care of their body and health, the usage of chemicals for long time may give changes genetically from this generation to the next one. Next generations may be more fatter and more likely having health problems. Do not stop doing sport at least to release those toxins! We try buying organic products which are more expensive but, we do not have the certainty they are clean of chemicals. The reason of this uncertainty is their different taste than the taste of those raised into a private garden or farm. What does it mean "organic"? Does not it mean no growth hormones and no genetically modified? Or, does it only mean no artificial substances and colors? But, "organic" surely does not mean no preservatives or not being pasteurized. We must look into the true meaning of this word "organic". What does the producer mean by this?

The world has been evolving and regressing in the same time. The food we eat today does not have the same quality as many years ago, even if it is manufactured at "higher standards". Certain foods are packaged to avoid bacteria and to make sure everything is handled in clean conditions. But, as an example, when the cheese stay packaged for more than a day, its taste changes. Additionally, it might contain different chemicals and preservatives and for sure it is pasteurized. Many countries at least from Europe, still sell cheese that is not packaged and not pasteurized. This way that cheese does not lose its nutrients and may also be tasted before buying it, for the client to know ahead the quality of the product he is purchasing. Some countries have a history of hundreds of years of selling unpackaged and unpasteurized cheese and nobody died because of this reason. Nowadays we say, the world is safer because we are eliminating the risk of bacteria in the food we buy, but the new food comes full of new different unhealthy substances which are worse and may cause uncured diseases when using these products for a long time. The meat from today that is sold at the organics section, it contains preservatives to keep it pink and nice in color on top, but inside is dark brown and it reveals its true quality. We consume the packaged products from supermarket but, our body is not so strong anymore naturally. We need to take different supplements to compensate the little nutrition today's food offers us. In the past, peasants were eating their food and had not taken any energizers to supplement it, but they were much stronger physically.

Before I arrived in United States, I had never drunk sweet milk or had eaten sweet sausage. I have never known before, that these "tasty" products exist. I am sure we can find these foods with sugar in composition in other countries as well. If they are not yet, they will get soon everywhere in the world. White sugar gives addiction very easy! In addition, I do not know where this idea comes from, to use honey or maple syrup in the sausage composition. I thought the sausage is made to be a regular dish to serve for hungriness, but not to be a desert to eat it for pleasure only. The worst fact is that many people feel that this sweet taste is the regular and the natural taste that a sausage should have. They are used to this type of taste and this is what they like. But, when a foreign person visits a different country, he finds these types of sweet products a little weird because he is not use to them. He grabs a pack of sausages from supermarket without reading the label to learn about its content, thinking this is just a regular pack of sausages. At home, he ends up throwing it in the trash and he will remain with no food for dinner. Or, he will like it so much that he will become addicted and he will go to buy more of those sausages. He will gain fat and his high blood sugar will get confused. The same happens with some types of milk. The regular milk has its natural sugar called lactose. But, certain milk products have additional sugar in composition. I wonder why??? Because we live into a modern world, we need to use modern products.

The new civilized world is fantastic! We have even got to peel the peach as the potatoes and bite in it like into an apple. It should be sweet at least but better sour than sorry. They could have adding some sugar in. I hope it stays just sour as it is. Hoping that the peach is hard because it needs more time to ripe, you buy it. But after couple of days, instead of becoming soft and juicy, it becomes soft, rotten and brown inside. Even that time, the outside skin of the peach is still nice in color, which is very interesting but surely not natural.

Remember when your grandmother was advising you to eat the skin of the apple because it contains a lot of vitamins. This is not the case nowadays. I personally must peel the skin out of the apple all the time because it can remain stuck in my throat. This much hard it is.

Moreover, these days, the apple skin may have a wax on it that cannot be washed off with simple soap. In the past, people use to wash the fruits with water only and they were not having healthy problems. In the civilized world, we need to learn to adjust and do not eat a fruit right out of the tree. It is not your own tree anymore. Buy the items from the store, wait before you go home and wash it with detergent. Many people have bad allergies because they did not wash the fruits with detergent. For better usage, leave it in the water with detergent for about 3 minutes and then rinse it off. Hopefully, that detergent will not enter in the fruit pulp and then in our body when the fruit is eaten. You are lucky if you have an allergy because of the chemicals in the fruits. At least you will know how to avoid getting sick and you will never forget to clean properly or peel the fruit. Unfortunately, there are people who do not have allergies or do not have any symptoms because of these chemicals that are used in fruits or vegetables. They are more at risk of cancer or bad health problems, because they may possible see the effects of the chemicals when it is too late. When a rash comes out on the skin, caused by a chemical, the body releases out the toxins caused by that chemical. This way our body has the ability to clean himself up or at least to signal us to take action. Another example of food full of chemicals or/and growth hormones is the tomato. This type of tomato is very woody and green in the middle, even if it may be red on the outside. Some types of chemicals made the tomato so bad for the system that we feel the effect right away. They give stomach problems as bloating and diarrhea. Or, there are tomatoes which have the skin so thick that it is hard to chew. But, they can cause even further problems which may not be observed as symptoms right away. Not to speak about the fact that the majority of the fruits and vegetables are picked up mostly green and ripe differently than their natural way or the store freeze them overnight and unfreeze them for the day. Wouldn't it be less work if they would not do that? Or, would not be more sales if the fruits would stay unfrozen? Personally, I would buy and eat more fruits if they had a good taste or be juicier and if they looked and were more natural. This is the reason for me to avoid buying and eating fruits for most of the times in the last years and this is not good at all. Bellow there are couple of images of good tomatoes in comparison with some worse ones.

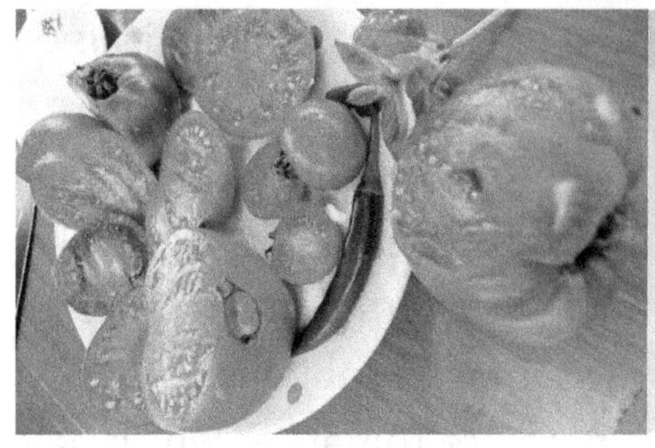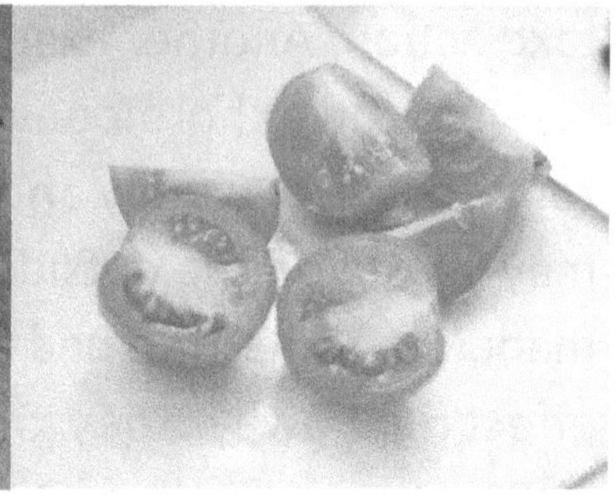

Natural Tomatoes
(not woody and not hard)

Tomatoes Artificially Treated
(woody and white inside)

Experts sustain that sometimes the tomatoes are given the red coloring by certain procedures, but they cannot give them the natural taste. Only the natural sun light is able to give them that good taste.

Strawberries are not anymore, the natural strawberries that we used to know and they still exist in some countries or at few rare farms. Strawberries should be much smaller, much softer and juicy. It is not a pleasure to try eating the outside layer of the strawberries only, when the inside is white, hard and not very edible. We pay for a certain quantity of strawberries and 70% we end up throwing in the trash. I feel cheated.

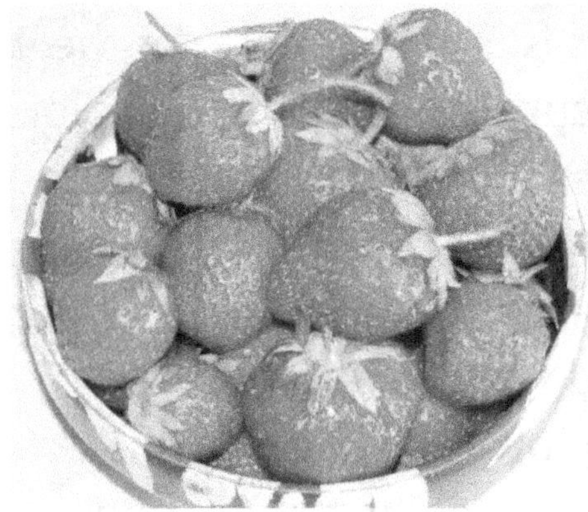

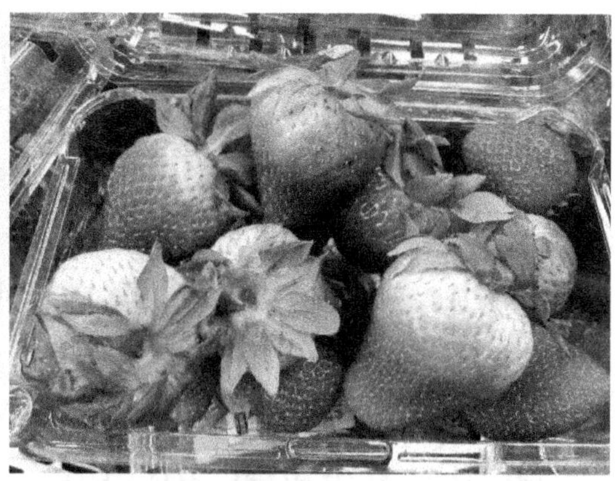

Natural Strawberries
(juicy, sweet, not woody)

Strawberries Artificially Treated
(white, hard inside, not sweet)

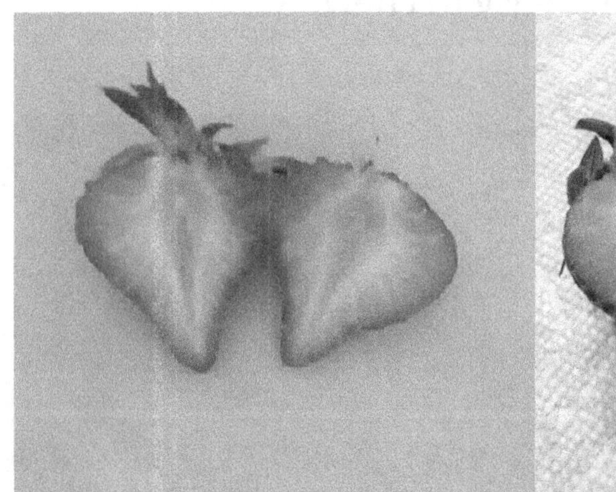

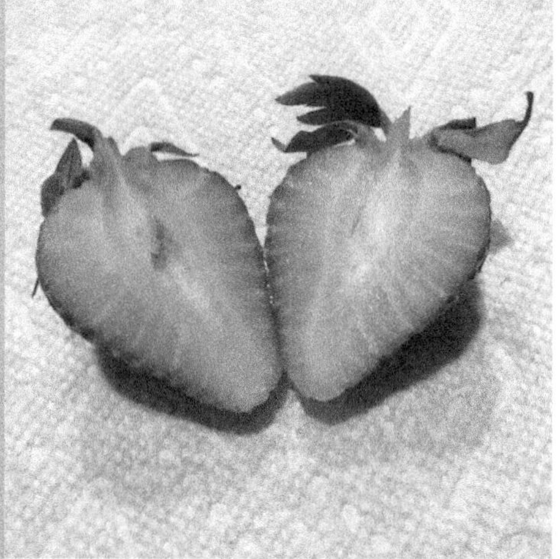

90% natural strawberries

90% artificial strawberries

As we see the above pictures, the artificial strawberries are not even fully ripe but they have already started to go bad. They are hard with no taste, when the natural ones are very ripe and they are still good with a fantastic taste. The natural strawberries are not woody and they are red everywhere inside. This is a natural color of the strawberries, natural size and consistency. The red color of the artificial ones, it is a fake color as you clearly see.

Another example is the grapes, as the evidence in the pictures bellow. Many grapes do not have seeds, fact that makes them easier to swallow. But, doesn't this mean those grapes are genetically modified? As other types of fruits, grapes contain chemicals or/and growth hormones, too. Natural grapes should be much smaller and their skin thinner and easy to chew.

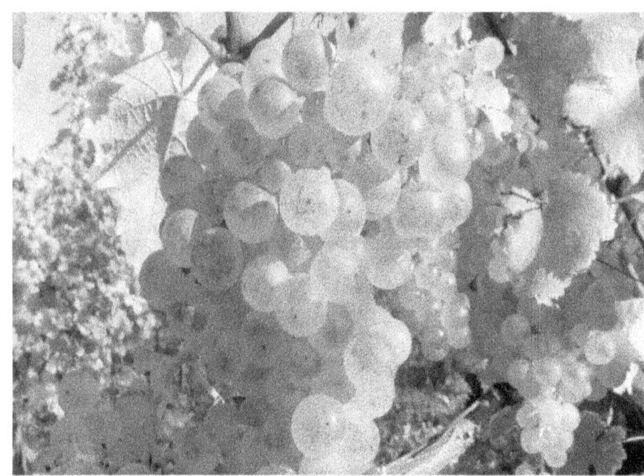
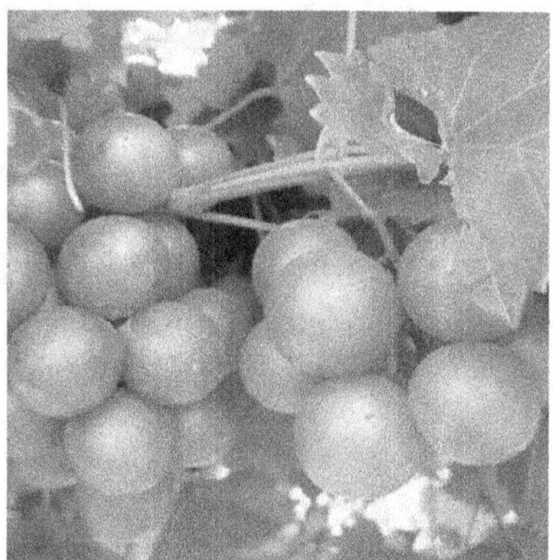

Natural Grapes   *Grapes Artificially Treated*
(always with seeds, thin skin)   *(way too big, unchewable skin)*

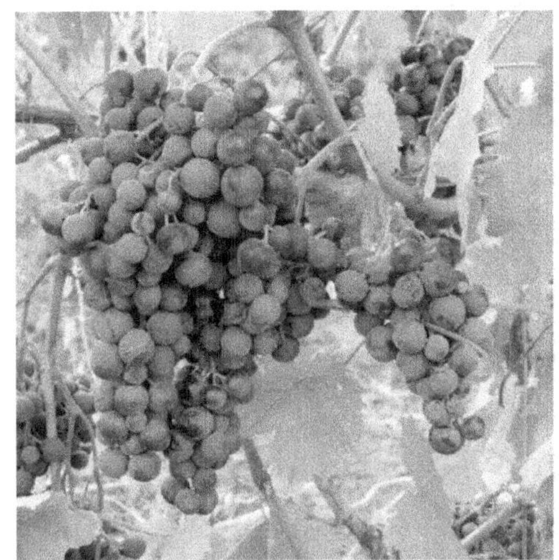

Natural Grapes

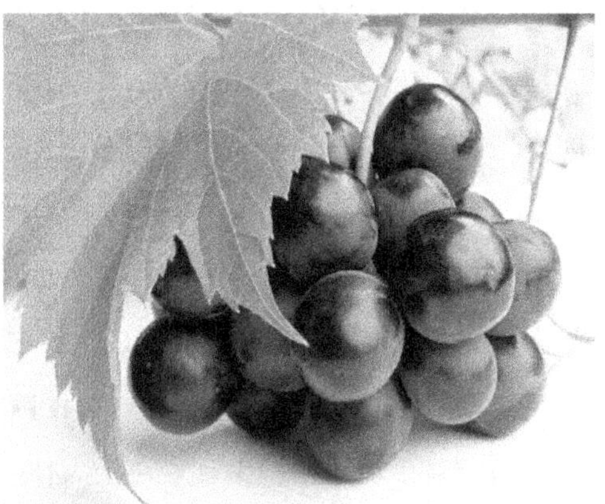

Grapes Artificially Treated

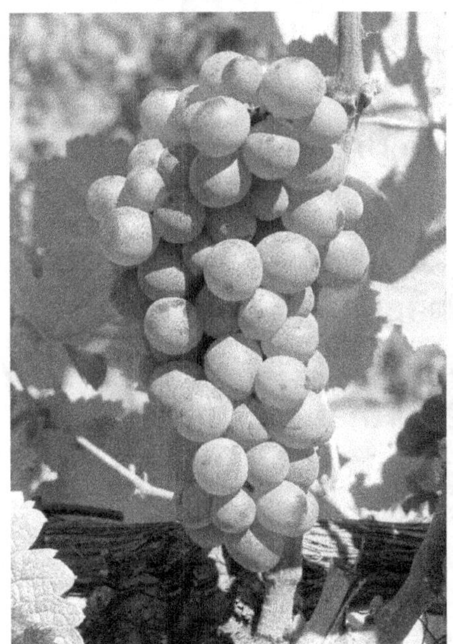

Natural Grapes

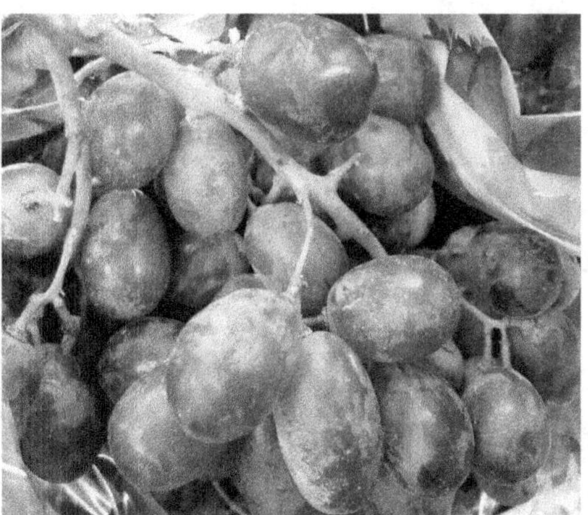

Grapes Artificially Treated

As we see, the modern black grapes look like plums and very glossy. These are surely not natural raised. The grapes today are sour in taste or way too sweet. Those which are sugary sweet, do not have a regular sweet taste. The taste is more like the sugar. I wonder why?

Another bad thing that brings toxins in the body is the enemy from the kitchen. As we see in different sources onto the internet, the **microwave oven** transforms the nutrients in carcinogens and lower very much the quality of the food we eat. Because we are in a rush most of the time, it is easier for us to use the microwave oven. Because of that, we need to find more alkaline sources to get rid of the acid accumulation. Moreover, we have to sweat much more and run much more to get rid of the toxins and implicitly of the cellulite.

The other bad thing that may happen to us is the usage of the **airconditioned unit**. Especially in U.S., the majority of the people use AC non-stop and they do not open the windows, at home, in the car, at work. Many people use the air from outside 1% of their time, only. Could you believe this? People who live in suburbs, start their usually day from the house (AC), going next into an indoor garage and in the car (AC) then, 2 minutes walking outdoor (where is not an indoor garage) from the car to the office building (AC), where they stay all day with no windows open (AC). In the best case, they end up using the outdoors 4 minutes per day only, back and forth. It is outrageous! In the majority institutions, the windows are built in such a way for not to be able to open. Even in the hospitals, the windows do not open at all. I may feel like into an incubator. All the patients are breathing a conditioned air which is coming from the pipes. When all those pipes are not very easy and very cheap to be cleaned and nobody is interested to do the effort and clean them, the people will breath the dusty air and whichever is growing in those pipes. In addition, the AC unit has a mash which needs to be periodically changed once per 3 months, otherwise it gets full of dirt. Usually the mash is not changed often enough or is not changed for years. Even it is changed in time, the mash is coated with certain chemicals to prevent the dust particles to get into the air. Those chemicals come off time to time and enter into the air we breathe. Moreover, if the AC unit is placed inside the apartment or the house and we do not open the windows enough, it might be another huge problem for our body. This air conditioned is drying the mucus in the nostrils and in the mouth. This will make the bacteria happy. Bacteria is around us all the time. It always depends about the strength of our immune system. When our immune system is weak, the bacteria will enter easier in our system and they will start the party. Not to mention about the skin dryness. I had lived in my country for 30 years. I had never used moisturizers for my skin. I did not need at all. My skin was permanently moist and smooth all those years. As soon as I got to U.S., after 1 week of my arrival, my skin got very dry. I thought I have a skin disease. Since then, it has been mandatory to use body lotion after each shower and every day for my skin not to itch. Otherwise, I scratch so much that my skin gets irritated. Is chlorine from the water a problem, AC which is blowing like crazy or a combination of both? The truth is, when the skin does not have the possibility to breathe regularly and it is not allowed to sweat enough to fulfill its natural role, it will not clean the body of free radicals and this will affect the health of our organs including the skin itself. The environment today obligates us to use the skin lotion all the time. The majority of the lotions contain certain substances which are not natural or may affect us overtime but we need to use them every day for the rest of our life.

All these said, we have to find time to clean and recover our body after the damages that the air conditioned does to us, too much quantity of certain substances in the water, certain soaps, lotions and detergents. How much do we need to sweat, how much do we need to run or eat alkaline, to manage all those toxins, this environment offers to us? And I didn't even mention about the headaches, colds, congestions or joint aches many people experiment when exposed to the cold conditioned air draft… But, there are people who really need cold conditioned air in the summer, especially if they live into a humid climate and not only. Logically, when a person has a thick adipose layer that covers him like a blanket and he is out of shape, it is hard for his body to adjust to the heat. Or, some people have a lot of hair on the body that keeps them warm. That is why we invented the AC for cold air. Instead changing our bodies to be more thinner and healthier to be able to adjust to the climate God offers to us, we have been changing the air or the environment around us. Even if the pipe air is not healthy, it may be used once in a while for a limited period of time. In general, anything that is moderately used, cannot kill us. Unfortunately, many people are suffering because of it. It is true, there are old people who suffer because of too much heat when is 90 degrees F (about 30 degrees C), too. But I wonder, the skinny 80 years old grandma who digs in her small outside garden at 80 degrees F (about 25 degrees C) and hates AC in her house because she says, it makes her not to be able to relax and the cold air drafts give her headaches, how healthy she might be??? What type of genetic has she inherited to be able to live better in the natural warm air? What type of food does she eat to keep her so strong? I know, you think there are no such people. Well, they exist. I have met them and they exist in big amount in certain parts of the world. They may just have said a prayer to God to be able to have these strong powers, but surely their physical work and eating habits have been helping them as well.

Not to forget about **air fresheners** that we use. Everywhere we can read about the bad damages they do to our body but we still use them. Certain people have allergies to them. Lucky them! This way their body tells them to avoid the air fresheners. They cause mucus dryness and breathing problems the same as the conditioned air does to us. I personally feel the way my throat dries out, it makes me cough and I even taste the chemical in my mouth when I am into an environment with that type of chemical and it is no window open or its concentration in the air is very strong. We may even read on their labels, when used in high quantity this product is toxic. But, the worst is when you do not have any symptom because of it. You would not know that it needs to be avoided. Even the air freshener that is used in the hospitals to kill viruses, it is harmful for us when used over the limit mentioned on the container. Do we use more than the safe limit? Here is another reason for an additional running session to get rid of these chemicals in our body!
To conclude, whatever kills the bugs, it may kill us, too.

This does not mean that we should live together with the bugs, elbow to elbow or skin to skin but, we should keep in mind that the chemicals that kill bugs, may kill us first and must be a way to use them less and be precautious. Bugs do not die so easy!

Dishwasher is a possible risk in the kitchen. It has both good and bad features. People in many countries do not use dishwasher. They have clean dishes all day long because they do not have to wait for a machine forever. In the civilized world we are much more lazier and this is the main reason we need a dishwasher. It also has some qualities when it washes the dishes at high water temperature but when it dries them may be an issue. The drops of water that evaporate in a closed space may form bacteria. When we dry something, it might be good to be dried at open air and not trapped in a space with no ventilation. Do not get me wrong. The dishwasher is good when we fill it with dishes very good prewashed by hand. The dishwasher does not have brushes to rub the dishes. The dishes must be washed really good with detergent by hand before put them inside the dishwasher. Otherwise, we risk to take them back full of remaining grease at their corners or with food on them. If we live couple of crumbs on a plate or on a fork, they will remain as dirt on them. It is even worse, during the process of drying, the dishwasher sticks that remaining food on the dish or fork and then, we have to rub the dish for a long time to take the dirt off. Wish you a happy rubbing! Would manufactories add couple of useful features to it and the dishwasher might be an effective machine. People from few countries are very used to the dishwasher as it is. They were born with it, they have been using it all their life and do not conceive the life without a dishwasher. For the rest of us, the dishwasher does not really help, it causes more trouble and it does not make sense.

I have mentioned earlier about the risks of the AC units and the dust or bacteria they may release. I am not surprised, so many people have allergies or breathing problems. Why do these allergens bother people that live in specific areas and do not bother when living in other areas on the globe? It may be too much pipe air we breathe every day. Another risk factor is pollution and who knows what particles do exist outdoors. In certain areas on the globe, people are screwed. Inside the building is "the artificial" air. Outside is pollution.

Moreover, in certain parts of the world we are private of natural **sun light** for the most part of the day if not for the whole day. This has surely an impact on our health and our stress level. Nowadays people encounter more stress in their life than the past generations. The stress is known to be one of many things who generates toxins in the body. Artificial light is another stress factor we are forced to use during the present days. Some office buildings are built like warehouses and not everybody has access to windows. 90% or even 100% of the day time, many people do not have access to the natural light. Because we need to have a job for earning some money, we must risk to get sick at any time. If a hospital midwife advises the mother to keep her new born child near the window where is more day light, so he will be able to have a healthy development and for gaining his immunity, why an adult would not need that, too? We are beings, we really need natural light. This type of light has something what the artificial light does not have.

During the last years, the sun is more dangerous for our skin than in the past. Actually, the ozone layer is the problem and not necessary the sun itself. We do not have much protection against the UV because the ozone layer is thinner. Why the ozone layer is thinner in certain parts of the world mostly? Should be the pollution or maybe different things that we are not even aware of. It is interesting that in my country, I needed to lay under the sun for 2 days to get some tan which in U.S. I get it in 1 hour. That is very effective! I am happy for the moment that I do not have to lose so much time with tanning. It works better than the tanning salons! Fabulous! But, is it healthy to get tan during a such short time? When I go running for 20 minutes only, dressed with a stripped tank top, I find myself already with tanned stripes on my skin. I have to use **sunscreen**... Many people use sunscreen all the time during the day, every day. For a simple trip to the store or when they just walk down the street, they apply sunscreen. This is a very weird world we live, in certain areas on the globe. Are you sure this sun screen is healthy to use it non-stop??? Does not this contain bad chemicals dangerous for our skin and body when used or inhaled them every day? Doesn't the sun screen trigger skin allergies or cancer more than the natural sun? Studies show that some sunscreens are safe. But, one thing is certain. When we inhale it, the sunscreen is toxic for sure and during the application on the skin inside a room, we inhale a lot of it. The overuse of anything is not healthy. The overuse of the sun is not healthy, nor the overuse of the sunscreen. Both help when we do not use them too much. There are studies who say that skin cancer does not come from the sun, as colon cancer does not come because we do not eat enough fibers or lung cancer does not come from too much smoking. I personally believe these reasons may contribute to illnesses, but I do agree that other reasons as the acid accumulation, are the main causes of this terrible disease. We let the researchers and medical professionals to help us with this acid.

People look for soaps and shampoos that are made mostly from natural ingredients. Unfortunately, there are also a lot of people who use the regular ones. Do you know that the most known brands use ingredients whose names start or include the group of letters "prop" and/or "prep"? There are specialists who say that these ingredients are carcinogens and people who get cancer, have a higher quantity of these types of substances in their body. Other studies say that cancer is a candida and that is why we may treat it with sodium bicarbonate. Whether these theories are true or not, the idea is that using a large quantity of chemicals, it develops free radicals and we may not sweat or eliminate enough toxins out of the body.

As I mentioned earlier, there are lucky people who develop allergies because of chemicals. This way the body releases the toxins. As an example, my daughter had really bad skin allergies in her first three years of life. We addressed many times this skin problem to the pediatrics and they said that nothing is wrong with her skin. Maybe they did not know how they can help for that skin condition. Usually allergies are very hard to diagnose and be certain of their cause. My daughter had redness all over her body, she was extremely itchy and full of rashes. She was scratching really bad during both nights and days and she had a very smelly discharge around her ears, soon after each time I gave her a bath. During a night, I thought she might die. I used the brand shampoos the doctor recommended. I thought she might have had these symptoms from the chlorine in the water. The chlorine might have contributed for sure but should I not wash her at all? I cannot do that. One day I stopped using soaps and shampoos. I started washing her with simple water only. I used olive oil to clean her scalp. She became better and better, in couple of months the skin started to clear up. The scalp became nice as well and there was no discharge around her ears anymore. Sometimes we just have to follow our instincts and get rid of the health issues this way. We need to survive. Good luck and have a less toxic life!

Chapter 9

Life of the Competitor
(last week before competition)

Bodybuilding is not an Olympic sport but it is a sport used by many people for different reasons. When doing it at a competition level, bodybuilding is a very complex sport. For good results, it involves good nutrition knowledge, correct exercise practice, commitment for daily serious training, cardio sessions involving different types of aerobic exercise, supplements dozes and times knowledge, focused mind and ambition. Like any other sport, it is helpful to keep in touch with a doctor and a massage therapist. Sometimes bodybuilding may become very dangerous, as all the sports are when done at a competition level. There are risks involved for developing health problems and if you are not careful, this may even bring death. Along with the doctor connection, you need to feel and know your own body and be ready at each moment to adjust your actions when your system reacts different than you were expected to. It is impossible for the doctor to stay with you 24 hours per day, especially because this is not a sport which brings money in most of the cases. Only a few top ones, at the professional level earn some and they may have a decent living. Moreover, it is good to be aware that few people did lose their life because they did not know when to stop or they exaggerated too much with dehydration or when they were doing other steps during the preparation for a competition. When everything is fine and we are able to control our diet, this sport is worth it. Looking back thankful that you won so many medals and trophies, it makes you feel confident in yourself with a strong balance forward in life.

This chapter is made for people who wish to compete and for the competitors who are at their first competitions and they are not sure about the last week preparation. Some bodybuilders start their preparation for the competition 6 months ahead of time. Usually, the professionals do this way and after those 6 months they may compete at multiple competitions one after another for a month. At that point, they should be in their best shape ever and they should take advantage of that by participating at more shows or at a full tournament. It is hard to stay in your best shape for a long time and it is not healthy at all. It is important to look perfect at the right hour and not 6 hours later, when the show is over. At these bodybuilding competitions, it even matters a difference of few hours and if you did a mistake related your supplements or water in the last week before the contest, you may lose one place right away. The professional competitors take a 3 months period of gaining more muscle mass, followed by another 3 months of losing fat. Now, it depends very much where are you starting from and what level of muscle mass and fat you have with 6 months before competition. If you are in a better shape, you may start with 4 months before, only. It also depends what type of competition you are participating at. Every type of contest and every Sports Federation have their rules. You have to know what the judges are looking for. As a general rule, they are looking for ripped muscles. The fat should be as minimum as possible to discover all the fibers. Does not matter what type of competition is, the fat should be at minimum. A higher volume of muscle mass is requested for the professional competitions in comparison with the amateur type competitions. Another important thing is the posture on the stage and the way you present yourself. Never have the shoulders dropped. All the muscle groups have to be permanently tensed. Do not forget about the legs when strain the upper body or reverse. Another quality of a good competitor is to be able to hide his defects. Everyone of us has defects but, for the time we are on the stage nobody has to see those defects. You may wonder how is it possible to do that, when you are dressed in swim suit only and you are in front of a large audience. As an example, for someone who has a thick waist, he always has to turn his abdominal area on the side or at 45 degrees. He must never stay straight, facing the whole abdomen width to the audience. Everybody has a disproportion more or less. Show the bigger triceps more than the other one, show the leg that seems to be more cut, etc. Of course, a competitor has to be proportional and have all the muscle groups developed the same. But, every human has slight differences between the left side and the right side of the body.

The females who compete at bodybuilding or into a category where a lot of muscle mass is requested, they have to be feminine as well. Their moves and presentation have to appear pleasant and feminine despite their muscle mass. On the other hand, the figure type categories are theoretically requested to have females which are not really cut, but just toned. The truth is the judges will always look for a body with a low proportion of fat. You still need to have good enough cuts in order to demonstrate that you do not have fat. That is why in a figure competition or bikini, the ones who are chosen for the first 3 positions are usually the girls with ripped muscles despite of the rules. They must also have a good proportion of the body.

You may find examples of muscle mass and losing fat diets in the chapters intended to serve for that purpose but here, you will find information about the last week diet before the competition. This last week is crucial and it can make a difference for everybody who competes. First of all, your body needs to be as lean as possible, with the minimum fat level, before starting the last week. It means that between the skin and the muscles we have water only and we do not have fat. This is the condition for this last week to be able to help with its "miracle transformation". In order to get rid of that water in between the skin and the muscles, bodybuilders or other competitors use some tricks. They also need to transfer some water into the muscle tissue to be pumped up on the stage and the skin should remain fixed on the muscle. If everything is correct done, they should feel the skin stretching around the muscles and nothing in between. This is just the feeling, because in reality the volume of the mass (fat + muscle) is less than during the off season when we do not have that feeling.

The first 3 days of the week, the competitor depletes his muscles of the carbohydrates. During the depletion he reduces the carbs amount to minimum and eat 90% lean protein. The other 10% should be the vegetables. Do not forget to eat vegetables for the first 3 days. Otherwise you may have bad constipation. The meals should be often, but do not eat too much for one time. Have a meal once per 2 or 3 hours with protein and vegetables to make sure the muscle mass does not atrophy. During the depletion, the water quantity should increase to wash out the whole system. In the first 3 days, we may drink 6 to 7 (240 ounces) liters of water. Some bodybuilders drink 9 or even 11 liters of water. I personally thing, this is way too much because we would force our kidneys. We need to think about our health, too and not just about a place on the podium. These three days we have to take lots of amino acids because during this short time the energy will come from the protein mostly. The protein powders are not recommended because they usually contain some carbohydrates. The competitors deplete or load for only 3 days because this is the limit when the body realizes the change. If this period is extended, the body will proceed with losing muscles when depleting or gaining fat when loading. Taking vitamins and minerals is crucial for the last week. During the first few days when we do not eat carbs, it is a must taking vitamins and minerals in a higher amount than usually. Otherwise our system will become weak and we might feel dizzy. Because of the high amount of water, we drink in 3 days only, the minerals and vitamins get flushed out of the body. The dose for each mineral or vitamin differs from one competitor to another. Someone may choose to take 1000 mg Calcium/day, 500 mg Magnesium/day, 1000 mg Vitamin C (3/day), Multivitamins 3/day, 500 mg Potassium. The last one is important for the last 3 days of the week mostly, during the carbs loading period. Potassium helps with introducing the water into the muscles. During the last 3 days before the competition, the individual increases the carbohydrates amount. He still has to eat proteins but at this point, the proteins are not so important as the carbs are. You do not build muscle mass anymore that time, you just maintain it and expand it with water. In the last 3 days before competition, the carbs we eat absorb all the water that is between the muscles and skin. That water and the glycogen from the carbs enter in the muscles and they expand very much. Because the muscles were depleted completely of glycogen during the first 3 days of the week, they are starving now. This is the reason that our muscles are absorbing much easier all the carbs we eat now, together with the water. These carbs have to still be complex carbs until few hours before the competition.

In the first 3 days of the week we drink a lot of water, followed by the next 3 days when the water is at minimum. We are shocking the body. When we suddenly stop giving him water, our body will retain more water because he is afraid he will not receive water anymore. But, it is important to retain water inside the muscles only. The carbs we ingest during the last 3 days will absorb the water that is retained in between the skin and the muscles. For those 3 days, we stop drinking additional water, not to fill the carbs with other new water than the one already existent in the body. Here, the potassium is also helping the water to be brought into the muscles only. This can be possible when we stop eating salt in the last 3 days, in the same time we stop drinking water.

If the trick with the water and the salt has a success, you will see much more fibers all over the body at the time of the competition.

In order to have toned and pumped muscles during the show, you have to eat some simple carbs 2 hours before the competition. It depends how dry you are for that time. If you are really dry, you may start eating simple carbs even 5 or 4 hours before. Do not start too early! You may become covered at the time of the competition. Simple carbs that you should eat couple of hours before the contest are chocolate, a cake, ice cream or anything you feel like eating that time to make you feel good and relaxed. Do not eat ice cream if you have lactose intolerance problems. Milk products may bloat you right away! Do not eat too much either! The stomach should remain flat but not straight. Little bit of simple carbs will be enough and they will help with both vascularization and a good tone of the muscles.

In a bodybuilding competition, the judges are looking for a good vascularization. The veins should pop up at the surface of the skin. This surely would place you with one step ahead in front of the other bodybuilders on the stage. For figure or bikini categories, the things stay different from this point of view. There is requested more femininity and elegance. It is a difference between a nice vasodilatation with healthy veins all over the body and having varicose veins. Varix are unhealthy veins that we do not want to have. They are actually a reason for punishment during the stage performance. The main condition for having a good vasodilatation is to be lean with no fat. The second condition is to get rid of the water in between the skin and the muscles and avoid to be puffy and covered. The third condition is to be relaxed and not to be stressed out. The stress raises the cortisol level and this may cover you. One thing is to be little nervous that helps you to focus and a different thing is being stressed out. An important tip of having a good vascularization is drinking a little bit of hard alcohol as vodka during the warm up in the back of the stage, with 20 minutes before entering in competition. Do not exaggerate with the alcohol! You do not want to get drunk and wobbly at the most important moment, for which you have been preparing so much. The night before competition, you may drink a glass of wine and then go to sleep early. The reason is that during the night you will wake up many times to urinate. The alcohol dehydrates and it helps to get rid of the remaining water from between the skin and muscle. The water from the wine will come out of your body, too. Be careful! Dehydration is very dangerous! If you stopped drinking water 3 days before competition, do not drink alcohol! In this case you are already dehydrated enough. Those 3 days are a long time when drinking just sips. This is very dangerous and I personally not recommend to stop completely the water with 3 days before. In the last 3 days, the competitor should only reduce the water very much for the body to notice the difference. This is the idea: the body has to see a sudden change in the water quantity we drink, that shocks the system and do not raise the aldosterone. After drinking around 7 liters of water during the first 3 days of the last week, we should reduce the water to 1 liter and 0.5 litters in the last 3 days of the last week. We could use that water for taking the vitamins and the necessary supplements. During the day of the competition we must have only sips of water

time to time. We do not add salt anyway and we do avoid completely the salty food. For this reason, our body cannot retain water. Some people use distilled water because this one does not contain salt and salts at all. I believe this is an exaggeration because it does not make a difference. At least it did not make for me.
On another hand, the high quantity of water from the first 3 days of the week, must not be reduced gradually before the competition day. After the first 3 days, we must drop suddenly the water quantity for the last 3 days. Otherwise the aldosterone may increase. This hormone retains the salt and water in the body and decrease the potassium level, because his natural role is to regulate the blood pressure. For the competition day, we need exactly the opposite. We need the potassium into the system as mentioned before, to help with bringing the water to the muscles. We need no water and salt in between the skin and the muscles. Theoretically, we do not have salt in the body at that point, but the water we drink it may contain some or some foods we eat as the eggs, contain naturally a lot of salt. This is a reason we should not gradually decrease the water. We do not need to assume any risk of becoming covered for those few minutes on the stage.

Another important thing that makes a difference is stop consuming dairy products in the last 2 weeks before competition. At least the last week you should not eat dairy products. Milk products make your body to retain water under the skin, you may become bloated as well and you will lose from the muscles definition.

Some people's muscles load with carbs much faster than others. These are usually the ones who have tendency to gain fat easier as the endomorph body types. They do not need more than 2 days of carbohydrates loading. Be careful! If you are not an endomorph, load for 3 days. Otherwise, you may remain flat and this would be such shame after all that work you have done during the last months. If your category enters on the stage Saturday morning, you may start the loading period on Wednesday evening.

The body may respond different to these tricks at each competition. A competitor may experiment the last week in different ways for each event and he sees where and what he should adjust. Only after a few competitions, a competitor may get used to the tricks that match his body. For example, some competitors have a loading period with salt during the first 3 days of the last week or for even 10 days. They cut the salt all of a sudden, for the last 3 days. This would be another shock for their system and the body would respond even better. They say, they become more ripped by doing so, for the day of the competition. I personally did not like to do a salt loading but each of us may choose different options for their preparation.

Let's say Saturday is the competition day. The following is an example of the last week diet.

Monday
water – 6 liters (throughout the day)
7:30 am – amino acids
8 am – 4 eggs omelet (2 yolks + 4 whites) + ham + mushrooms
10 am – chicken + green beans pods + lettuce
12 pm – amino acids
2 pm – chicken + green beans pods + lettuce
4 pm – nuts
6 pm – fish(no breading on top) + steamed kale
8 pm – amino acids
10 pm – fish + steamed kale
3 am – amino acids

Tuesday
water – 7 liters (throughout the day)
7:30 am – amino acids
8 am – 4 eggs (2 yolks only) + avocado + red pepper
10 am – beef + steamed spinach
12 pm – amino acids

2 pm – beef + steamed spinach
4 pm – nuts
6 pm – shrimp (1 bowl) + homemade tomato sauce (no sugar)
8 pm – amino acids
10 pm – 4 egg whites + tomato
3 am – amino acids

<u>Wednesday</u>
water – 7 liters (throughout the day)
7:30 am – amino acids
8 am – 4 eggs (2 yolks) + ham + olives + radishes
10 am – chicken + avocado + tomato
12 pm – amino acids
2 pm – chicken + lettuce
4 pm – chicken + green beans pods + lettuce
6 pm – amino acids
8 pm – fish (no breading on top) + veggies
10 pm – fish + veggies
3 am – amino acids

<u>Thursday</u>
1 liter water (throughout the day), no salt
7: 30 am – amino acids
8 am – firm (or dry) oatmeal + raisins (20)
10 am – 2 eggs + rice cakes (no salt) + avocado + radish
12 pm – rice + beef + steamed bean pods

2 pm – amino acids
4 pm – rice + beef + steamed veggies
6 pm – dried fruits
8 pm – beef + quinoa
10 pm – nuts
3 am – amino acids

Friday
0.5 liters water (only sips throughout the day), no salt
7:30 am – amino acids
8 am – rice + raisins
10 am – 2 eggs omelet + spinach + rice cakes
12 pm – pasta + olive oil + shrimp + asparagus
2 pm – amino acids
4 pm – pasta + olive oil + shrimp + asparagus
6 pm – dried fruits
8 pm – rice + chicken
10 pm – nuts
3 pm – amino acids

Saturday
sips of water only, no salt
7:30 am – amino acids
8 am – 2 eggs + 1 slice bread(preferably unsalted) +
butter + avocado + coffee(no milk or cream)
10 am – potatoes (hard cooked) or rice/rice cakes
12 pm/1 pm - chocolate (or a dessert)

2 pm – COMPETITION
4 pm – any food you wish

During the loading period we have to eat drier food mostly. That food has to be able to absorb the water from between the skin and the muscles. We have to avoid the fresh fruits because they contain a lot of water. For example, the rice or pasta should not be boiled too long. They must stay firm and not become mushy.

In the fourth day of the last week, do not start eating suddenly too much quantity of carbohydrates and food, unless you are an ectomorph. Otherwise, eat natural using normal portions for you. Be patient. You are on the right path towards the success. The muscles will load progressively in those 3 days and you will stay with your stomach flat. We do not want to have a protruding belly that would be impossible to pull in at the time of the competition or you may even have an indigestion. During the loading period, the proteins are helping first of all for not experiencing diarrhea and for having balanced meals. When we eat mostly carbs, vegetables and dried fruits too much but not proteins with it during the day, we may have serious indigestion and we may lose from the muscle mass. For example, dried fruits contain a lot of potassium and magnesium. We have to be careful, when we have too much or too little potassium and magnesium, it may occur bad muscular cramps. When we have too much potassium, we may have diarrhea. Our body is very sensitives to all these details. A competitor has to learn by himself the body reactions and form his own style of preparation for competitions. Even if he has a pretty big experience with this, every competition may be different and his body may not react the same way. Do not be disappointed if the tricks did not work out for you at some competitions. After each contest you will become more experienced and each time you are on the stage or go through a contest preparation, it teaches you something good. You will learn more and more from all the contests you go through. By participating only, you can develop your own techniques as well as your muscle growth which gets more mature over time.

The workouts for the last week should be little different than the regular weeks during the preparation. Bellow you can see the way a competitor should exercise during the last week before competition. During the first 3 days we must deplete of the glycogen, all the muscles in the body. The last 3 days, we have to load the muscles with glycogen and water.

The purpose for these first 3 days is not to build muscles anymore. We need to get rid of the glycogen only. That means we do not have to use the heaviest weights ever or break any record these days. We will be weaker anyway, especially on Tuesday or Wednesday. We must be careful and do not have any accident of the lower back or certain joints and muscles issues.

<u>Monday</u>
Legs (hamstrings + quadriceps + calves), Abs
running (or any aerobic)

<u>Tuesday</u>
Chest, Back
running (or any aerobic)

<u>Wednesday</u>
Arms (triceps + biceps), shoulders
running (or any aerobic)

<u>Thursday, Friday, Saturday</u>
No exercise

   The competitions with lots of participants, have 2 or even 3 days of competition. Usually there are 2 competitional days. The first day is for the qualifications when competitors are seen more or less on the stage, so the referees could determine the participants who are fit for the final. The first 6 competitors or the first 10 ones, go further to compete on the last day when is the final.

In this case, the last week preparation should be about the same. The qualification day would fall on the second day of the carbohydrates loading. You should be loaded enough for that competition stage. You should not load the muscles with simple carbohydrates as chocolate for the qualification day. Continue to load slowly. If you did the right diets and workouts for the entire period of 3 months before, you should be now pretty ripped anyway and you will surely qualify for the final.

The first 3 days of the week we need to exercise smart to deplete all the glycogen out of the muscles. We need to work the muscles from all different angles. We must increase the numbers of the repetitions for the purpose of depleting the muscles. We may do between 10 to 15 reps per set. The workout has to lean towards a cardio weight lifting version. Running or any other aerobic exercise is good to be done. These help the depletion process, as well. Those days, we are eating protein only, but the muscles still have the glycogen from the carbs that we have ingested before the last week. By Wednesday evening, all the muscles in our body should be depleted and very hungry of energy. Do not forget to take plenty of vitamins and minerals to make sure you do not get too weak. Thursday morning starts the loading period. This is the reason we stop exercising. We need to allow the muscles to recover nicely and expand little by little. We suppose to see the muscles enlarging in volume hour after hour. We need to have patience and do not eat too much at once. Our muscles get happy and our brain gets very happy that we finally give them carbohydrates. We should still have to be disciplined by keeping under control the food quantity we eat. We do not have to relax too much, even if we might have a tendency of doing so, for these last days. These carbs have to go into the muscles. We need to give them some help by posing a lot and by flexing them. This way the glycogen from carbs will know better the path towards all the fibers. Posing and flexing the muscles is very important to be done more during the last 3 days before the competition. We need to sweat when posing and flexing for 15, 20 or 30 minutes every day. Those who compete in bodybuilding, they may use these 20 minutes to rehearse their free music program for many times. This will be the only exercise for these days. If possible, try to keep a warm temperature in the room. The muscles function better at a higher temperature environment and you will be able to get rid of all the water retention much easier. It is not recommended to lift weights during the last days. The muscles will not load and you will be thin with no muscles and tone at the show. If only you believe you still have some water retention between the muscles and the skin, you may run one time in the last day before the competition. Do not overdo it because the muscles have to load with glycogen.

During the 30 minutes before the competition, you should already have in the muscles the glycogen from the simple carbs you have just eaten. Slowly, we need to start that warm up before entering on the stage. Do not wear you out! Do not lift heavy weights that time! You only need to flex the muscles to have a tone and pump the blood for a good vascularization. If you still have a lot of fat at the point, the pumping will not help the muscles or the veins to be seen. Hopefully the show room will not have cold conditioned air. When it is too cold, the muscles cannot dilate good and the veins cannot come at the surface. All the tissues squeeze and you may look common. If you start sweating at that warm up, it is a good sign. Luckily there are reflector lights on the stage which make you stay hot. In the back of the stage you may warm up doing couple of exercises with the simple barbell only or some easy dumbbells. A few contest organizers do not even bring any small weights for the back of the stage. The organizers are not all the time ex competitors. They may not know the importance of these details. This should not scare you. You may warm up by flexing your muscles only. Competitors could warm up together by pulling (for back) and pushing (for chest) each other or using a towel. It is helpful if you have a friend with you. The muscles should not be too pumped, especially the legs. When they are too hard and round, the referees will not be able to see properly all the cuts you may have. The muscles should remain soft but toned. Posing on the stage is exhausting. You need energy left for the 5 or 20 minutes when you are on the stage. You need to keep all your muscle groups flexed in continue for the whole time you are on the stage. I had personally looked very small and thin when I had clothes on me or in the back of the stage in comparison with the majority of the competitors. On the stage everything was the opposite. Lucky me!

An experienced competitor has different tricks he may do on the stage. During the show there are a lot of reflector lights on the stage. It is hard to see the people in the audience. You are barely seeing the referees. At some competitions, they use different reflectors in certain parts of the stage which may have stronger light. When possible, you should look to stay in front of those stronger lights. This way, your fiber cuts and details can be perfectly seen. When you are in a shadow, you will look smooth. This is an advantage of the modern world. The reflector lights on the stage do not give any problems to the competitors. They are usually very well placed.

In the past and sometimes today, competitors use a

special dark cream on the body. The body details can be seen better on the dark surface. The black people have an advantage. The white guy has to make sure his cream does not drain on his body when he sweats during the show. That would not look good at all. Luckily the last few years, there are spraying machines that people use to blow the special cream very uniform all over the body. Those creams are more effective, but usually quite expensive, too. They do not drain when in contact with the perspiration. Actually, they wash out of the body after 2 or 3 weeks only.

The first month after the competition is the main proper period for gaining muscle mass. During that time, our muscles are able to absorb a lot and to grow. If we continue to eat permitted foods mostly and do not exaggerate with the simple carbs and bad oils, we will build very fast qualitative muscles during this time. After the show, many competitors eat a lot and without limits. Mentally they believe that time is the best for doing mistakes. They cover themselves very fast and after 3 days, they start gaining fat. After one month they become like a big blob of fat, a huge soft and shaky mass. During their off season, they should compete for sumo. This is not healthy first of all. Secondly, they do not look good and their skin stretches very much. That will affect the quality of their skin after few years of competitions, especially after the age of 45 or 50. Thirdly, they must start losing that much fat again in a little while, which is not quite easy work to do. Moreover, these repetitive changes in weight, trigger also a change in the metabolism and after years, our body would need more and more strict and difficult diets in order to look at least decent.

It is very important to be in good health to experiment the last week before the contest. Do not try these methods if you have chronic illnesses or kidneys issues. The last week strains the body very much and the individual has to be perfectly healthy for his body to answer the way it is written in books.

Disclaimer:

The content of this book serves as informational purpose only. This book is not intended to offer information for diagnosis or treatment of a medical condition. The opinions expressed in this writing are those of the author. Before using the information in this book please ask the opinion of a physician or a health care professional. **Do not** take any decision about your health, before asking the advice of a health care professional. This book does not recommend self-management of health issues. The information in this book including nutritional supplements and doses should not be considered as a substitute for the advice from a healthcare professional. The publisher and the author are not responsible for any specific health or allergy needs that may require medical supervision and are not liable for any damages or negative consequences from any treatment, action, application or preparation to any person reading or following the information in this book. This book is made by an ex competitor and personal trainer but not a physician or a doctor. The book may mention healing approaches that are experimental and may not be approved by FDA. Thank you.

About the Author

Being surrounded by competitors and many people who enjoy doing a sport and looking good, I thought having knowledge about nutrition and exercise is something natural and common. I thought everybody around have the minimum information in this field. But later, I have discovered there are more people than I expected, who do not know details about exercise and healthy eating habits. I have decided to do this book for sharing with you the information I have been gathered during my competitions years and after that period. I do not compete anymore because my life took a different path and it is not enough time to focus mostly on the details that a competitor's life would involve. In addition, sometimes the risks may overcome the benefits when we do this sport at a competition level for a too long time. Off course, I do not regret I competed because that was one of the most beautiful periods of my life, but like every good and beautiful thing in life, also this one had to have an end. Sometimes we have to know when to stop because there are other things during a life span that are nice to discover and good to be done. Like any other sport done at a competition level, this one involves certain risks, as well. For me it had an impact on my joints. That was because of too much running on the concrete. When others had used much more supplements to lose weight and they had not done too much physical effort, I was just running 2 times per day and at one competition I ran 3 times per day for losing the adipose layer. I guess, I chose the hardest way which was not necessary the smartest way because it did not do good for my knees and ankles. In addition, when you over train, your body stop responding the way you wish, because he is too exhausted. I did mistakes and I learned from them. My knees were hurting bad in the night or when I was sitting

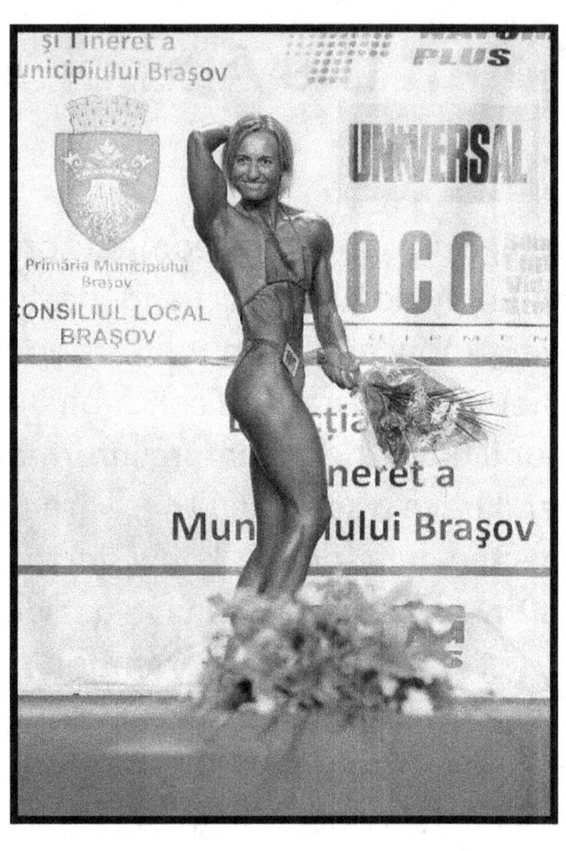

for few hours in the same position at work, but not when I was running. I needed about 2 or 3 years to heal and take MSM with glucosamine, chondroitin and others on and off, to nourish my knee cartilage and heal completely. Now I am running once per day sometimes or 3 times per week some other times and I have not been feeling any pain for many years. It is amazing what MSM can do.

I have only started going to the gym for the first time in my life, in the 3rd year of my college, at the age of 20. Me and my roommate decided to go. She gave up after 2 months and I continued. I remember she was saying about her childhood. She had not taken any supplements as vitamins and minerals and she had not have patience to eat. She told me, when she was a child, she used to grab one slice of bread with a spread on it and run outside to play for the whole day. It is very important to eat properly when you are a child and have a diverse nutrition in order to have strength and energy when you grow up. It is interesting but true that the regular vitamin and mineral intake during the childhood, it really makes a difference later on in life and gives you physical strength and health after years. When I was a child, my grandparents gave me vitamins almost every day and after years I have been seeing the results. After 2 months going to the gym, I saw that I like it a lot and I could see my muscles developing slowly. In fact, I have always wanted to build muscles since my childhood days in order to have a decent shape, but I did not know the way this can be done. I did not wish to exaggerate in these sense, either and become too manly. My style is more feminine.

By the time I finished my Master degree, I have already had my first competition. It was the first and the last one when I did not win a medal. It was a total failure. I was placed the 4th. This is the worst place ever. I would have been better of with the 5th place. When you know you are so close to the podium and you are actually not on it … I made sure all my future competitions were not a waste. From then on, everything was calculated for the next competitional preparations. The daily protein intake, the water quantity, the supplements and the last week. Everything came out good and my body responded exactly as it was supposed to, the way I predicted. I started to learn my body reactions. I was reading different sources about bodybuilding contest preparations. I was able to combine the different type of diets and choose from each of them, the part that fitted my body only. I did also mistakes at each competition, but they were minor and the success did not go around me. For every competition, my goal was to win a place on the podium. I did not even hope that I may take the first place. I guess this was one of my mistakes. If I was about to focus more on winning the first place, I would have gained more. I have won, what I focused on. But, I cannot be too sad about this.

Otherwise I made enough mistake. For example, I have run too much when I prepared for a contest. I ran two times per day, every day for the whole period of 2.5 months or 3 months and I tried to stay physically active throughout the day. I was afraid I cannot lose in time the adipose layer I had. I have never been fat, but when you compete the expectations are different. Your body has to be very lean. By running so much I may have lost a lot of muscle mass. At the time of the contest I was very ripped but I have never had a lot of muscle mass. I knew the main important thing was to be ripped. That put me indeed, in front of the other competitors.

An unhappy moment was when being on a strict diet, I tried doing squats with no belt and one of the vertebras from my lower back, got out of its regular spot. For the next 2 or 3 weeks I barely could bend on top of the sink to wash my face. I had a sharp pain to my lower back when I did so. It was very painful for me to tie my shoe laces. I could walk slowly but I felt at each step sharp pain at the same area. I knew I have to do something as soon as possible. I had to move back in place my vertebra, without waiting for too long. I believed that if I waited for many months with my vertebra out of its regular spot, it will be hard to put it back in place mechanically. I could not even have conceived to do a surgery. That should be avoided as long as we can. Nowadays, there are therapists that can help you mechanically with this type of issues. Even if you are at the point that you cannot walk at all, certain therapists are able to help you and avoid the risky surgery. The unbearable pain may push you to run quickly to the surgeon but better bear for a little while and try going to the different types of therapists and do their procedures. Unfortunately, in U.S.A. therapists do not do the 10 procedures that

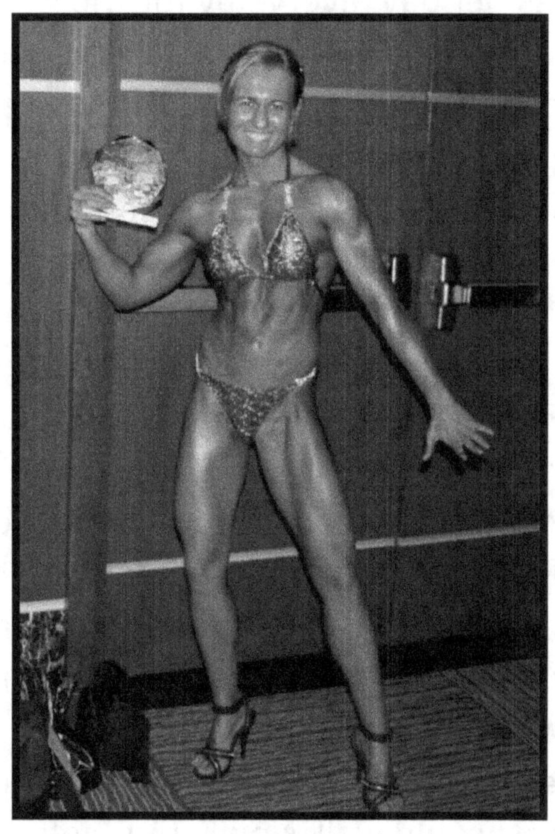

are done in my country for this matter, but they have other techniques which are helpful and are not so risky as a surgery.

My back pain was bad but the fear that my spine will

form this way if I do not rearrange my vertebra soon, it was worse. I tried to put it back mechanically. I massaged by myself many times per day the spot. It was the vertebra L4 or some of the L ones. I tried to push it back in place with my fingers. It did not work. I tried doing certain movements and stretching to help. That vertebra was still out of place. I was still going to the gym and work my upper body only as much as I could and using mostly the machines. Sometimes I stayed hung down of a barbell that was placed high up. I asked my friend to grab my lower body and pull it down. After about 4 attempts done over couple of weeks, I felt and heard my vertebra sliding into his original place. I was lucky! After 3 days of more pain than before and inflammation at the lumbers area, I was healed. Huh!

Doing squats with no belt during a low carb diet, I cannot call it a mistake. It was a misfortune. It could have happened anyway. It is interesting that the moment it happened, I was lifting very light weight. This did not happen when I have lifted heavy. Lifting weights with the barbell on your traps is the most effective exercise for legs but it also involves risks. The weight is pressing the spine and for sure after years of doing squats, more likely it will affect the back bone. On another hand, there are many people who do not even do sport or any exercise and have problems with their back. The difference is, the ones who do exercise, look good and stimulate their blood to flow better, stimulate the lymphatic system to release out the free radicals and their chances of healing are higher.

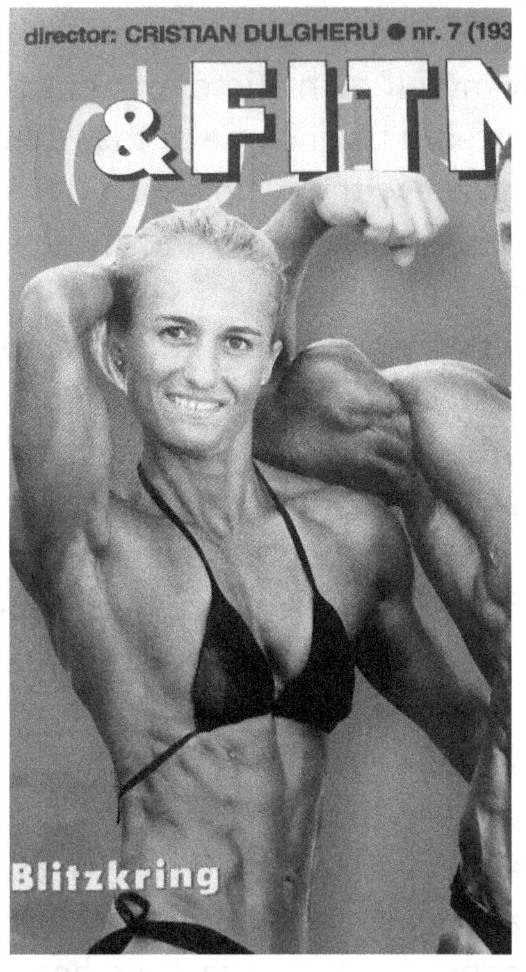

   Looking back at the way I did my workouts, there are certain things that I would improve if could turn back in time. It is known that legs muscles develop harder than the upper body. Many people do not even work much their legs because it is harder to develop them. They just quit and work on the other body parts which present a faster development. This is the reason they are not proportional. I have worked out my legs one time per week as all other muscle groups but this was a mistake on my behalf. I should have had weeks with 2 workouts for legs per week. My legs muscles needed to develop much more. I was told by women, masters of this sport that I had a very good proportion on the stage. I believe that was because I had a thin waist, an upper body and lower body about the same length. But now I know, if I could have had more mass built on my legs as a female, I would have won each competition with no problems. For a female, it is harder to have both muscle mass and definition of the legs in the same time. She has the estrogen which stays in the way. I have chosen to be ripped and lose some of my muscle mass during the preparation but ensure a place of the first three. I had competitors around me on the stage with much more muscle mass but they were not so ripped. They placed themselves towards the last places.

One of the mistakes I did during my last week before a certain competition was that I had completely stopped drinking water for those 3 days before it. As explained in the last chapter, in order to become very defined at the time of the contest we need to have sips of water only, within 72 hours before going on the stage or reduce the water at a minimum for the body to feel the difference in the water quantity. Stopping completely the water intake is very dangerous. It is a mistake that I have done. Usually, I was reducing the water from the 6 and 7 liters in the first 3 days of that week, to 1 liter and 0.5 liters for the last 3 days. During the last week of one of my competitions, I stopped drinking water completely for the last 3 days meaning that I did drink couple of sips per day only and that was all. I have exaggerated. This made me too dehydrated and during the last night before the competition, I felt little weird and way too weak than usual for that stage. That moment I was not concerned anymore about the contest. I started drinking water. I believe I had drunk 1 liter in 5 minutes despite the following day's results. At the contest I came on the 3rd place anyway but for me, it was a failure. I could have done much better if I had not dehydrated myself so much. This is one of the many mistakes that competitors may do and they are forced to learn to be a doctor of themselves. A doctor cannot guard you at every hour and during the nights. We have to be aware of our own body reactions and must have lots of knowledge before starting to compete.

I had stress sometimes, during my life. I guess nobody can completely go around stress. When someone has to get ready for a competition, this factor may influence the ability to focus and the body may not answer the regular way. My advice is, for the time periods when you are stress out, do not prepare for a competition. Before a contest, during my preparation for one of my bodybuilding National Championships, I did both strenuous physical activity and I encountered stress situation. As a result, during my workouts, my left arm was swelling up and it had an unusual tone to it. I did not

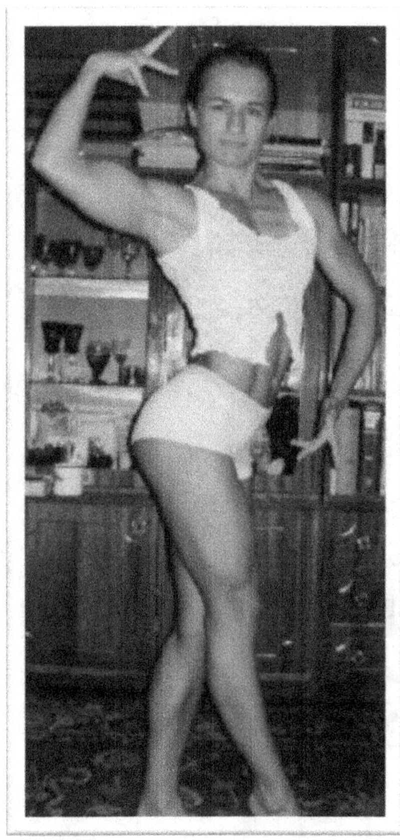

have other symptoms, but I understood that something is not right. When I was running, I had numbness sometimes and tingling to that hand. I have been to many doctors for that problem but all my tests results came out good. I knew that the only reason for my symptoms is together the stress and too much physical effort. I stopped doing any running or lifting weights for one month. It is almost impossible to eliminate the stress in couple of days. It takes time. When I restarted to get ready for the same competition, there was left 1 month only before the big day. I had to take it easy during my workouts and running. At the contest I won the 2nd place and the title of Bodybuilding National Vice Champion. Many people congratulated me and they said I looked good for the contest, but I have personally seen myself kind of dried out inside the muscles, too. Everything is good when the finish line is good.

With every competition I have gained more experience. The preparation steps and the last week before competitions were going more natural and easy. After all, I have been continuing to learn about nutrition and try to carry on a healthy life. Every day we may encounter new situations because our body changes over time and we have to adapt.

During my 3 months diet before the competition, I had eaten very strict and calculated all the steps with accuracy. I took it very seriously and I pushed myself to continue the diet. I counted the protein grams every day but I did this by nature. It was not a struggle to manage my daily nutrition. I used that eating mistake one time per week, Sunday and that recovered my energy in the muscle and for the brain.

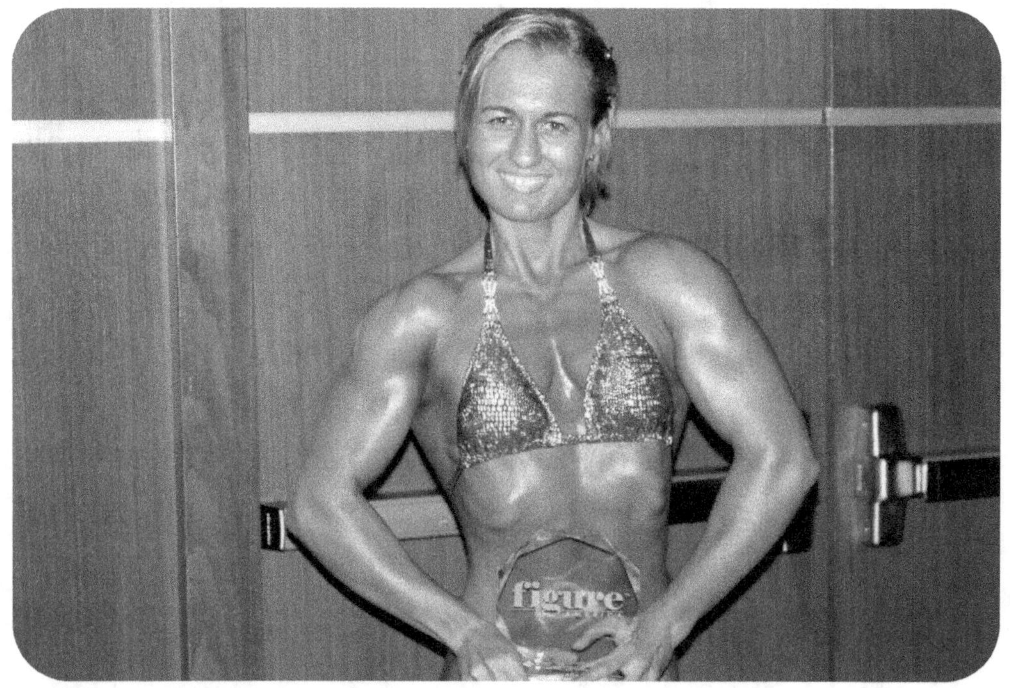

At each stage, I stopped eating certain types of foods. For example, I took out of my diet the dairy products with 1 month before the contest because they retain water and I was looking more covered when using them. I could have stopped using milk little later but for that time, I preferred to stop it earlier for mental encouragement. Little by little I had also stopped eating other foods. In the last 3 weeks, I was eating only the few basic products from each food category.

What should I have done to lose fat faster? I could have stopped adding salt on my food. I did not do that. I preferred to have a little longer diet but using salt. I like salty foods and it is very hard without it. Luckily, I usually have a low blood pressure and I could include salt in my diet. Plus, when I had eaten the chicken breast or boiled beef, it was very hard to swallow them. They are very dry and the salt was the one who helped me. I could have used olive oil or the healthy oils, but that would have been too greasy for my taste. Moreover, the olive oil also contains little saturated fat and using it in a high amount every day before a competition, I believed it might have a negative impact for my preparation. Olive oil is known to be healthy when used as dressing, but I still did not trust using it for those weeks only.

My diets brought results and many times I finished my losing fat process even too early. I was done with the fat loss with 3 weeks before competition. Those times I was thinking, now what should I do till the competition is here? During my last 3 weeks, I had just maintained and polished my body. Maybe if I had not finished with losing the fat so quickly, it could have remained more muscle mass, too. I wanted to make sure I got ripped in time and I was not too late with my diet progress.

The losing fat process went quite well each time but getting ready so many times for competition involved a change of my metabolism. Like any other competitor who keeps many severe diets on and off, the body answers by lowering the metabolism. Year after year, we have to keep diets more and more severe for losing fat. We have to cut more out from the food quantity we eat and cut out foods which did not get us fat in the past, but now our body feels that they have a too high glycemic index for our present metabolism.

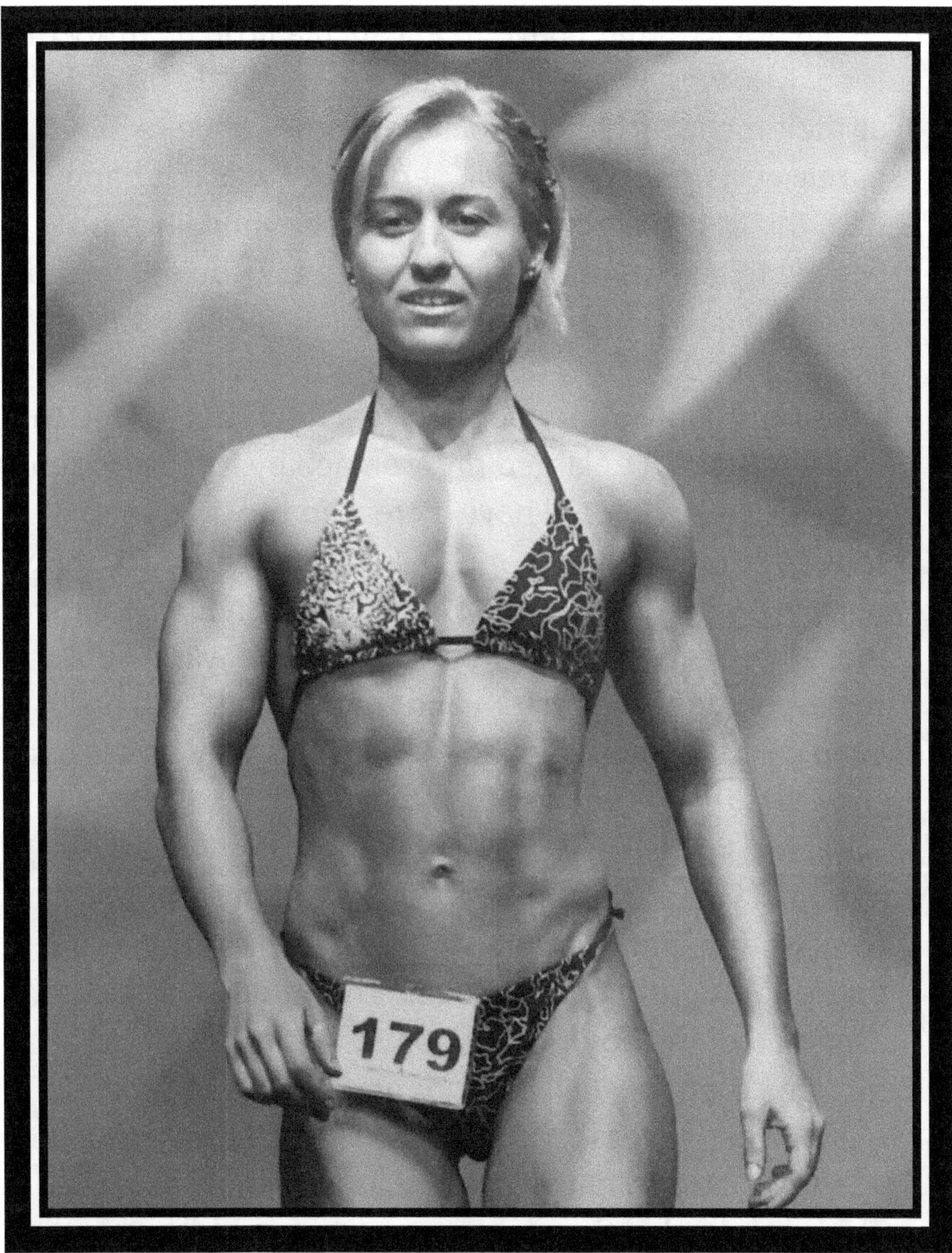
179

I did not like that I have to eat such a little quantity of food. Me, who I barely could have eaten little bit of food at the time I started bodybuilding, now I have to avoid eating certain foods to look perfect…. I was not happy with this at all. When I had started bodybuilding and wished to gain as much muscle mass as I could, I forced myself to eat 4 eggs at one meal or bigger portions of rice and food. For my body weight, that was too much of a quantity. Only after about 10 years, I have realized that was a mistake. I enlarged my stomach by forcing so much food inside it. I should have increased the amount of food little bit but not so much. I do not even know if my body was able to process so much food and form muscle mass. I believe that a quarter of that food was just released out of the system and that was all. I did not even gain fat. I have gained muscles but very slowly over the years that were passing by.

When I was almost 30 years old, I had my last competition and I was placed the 2nd. This one was a figure competition in Las Vegas. That time I was kind of ashamed of my boyfriend who was eating less food quantity than me. I was wondering, how is he able to manage eating less food quantity when he was double in size than me and having a lot of muscle mass as well. Then, I started eating the same portion and the same type of food as he did. At the time we both finished our dinner, he was fine, but I was really hungry and this way I struggled to go to bed in the evening. I figured my stomach is too large and I needed to get back at my regular stomach size

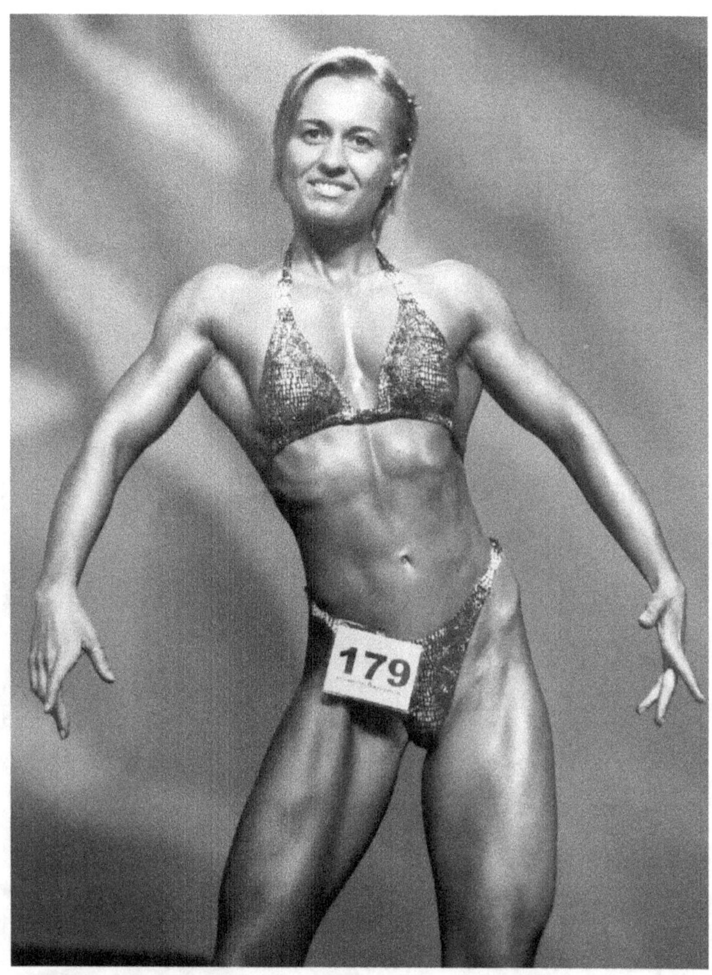

I had, when I was 20 years old and I had started bodybuilding. At 20 years of age I could have eaten any type of food at any hour and half of bread a day and I did not increased too much the adipose layer. I was considered too skinny for that age.

I am going to tell you my partner's secret for that time. He used to eat his regular meal at the regular size. But, he completed his dinner with a regular half of a chocolate cake. This is the reason he was not hungry anymore after his regular dinner. When he was coming at home with a full round cake, I thought it is his birthday and we have to celebrate. This was not true. It was no event and no birthday to celebrate. He finished the cake in 2 or maximum 3 days all by himself and he was still in a very good shape. How fortunate he is to have such genetics. Such a high quantity of simple carbs and he has not really got fat.

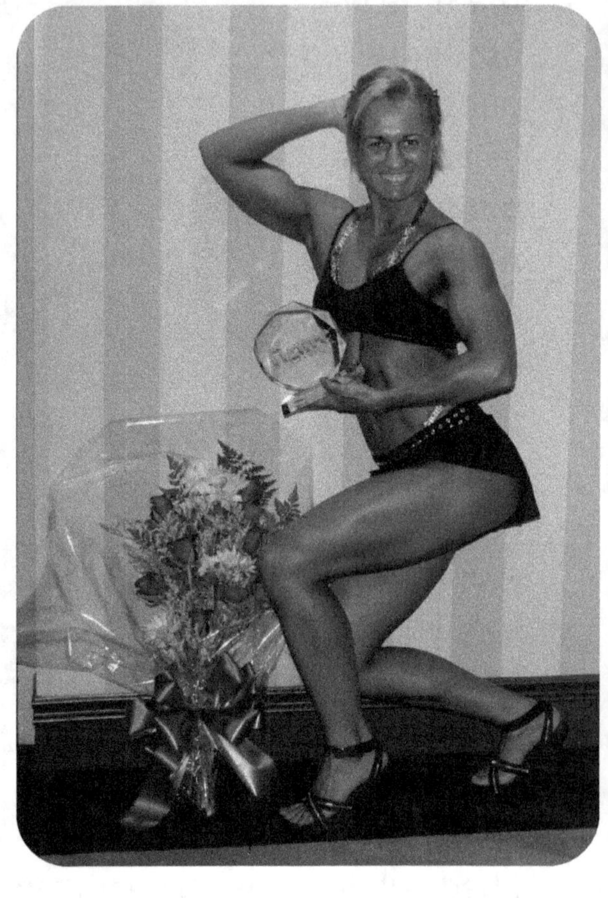

Speaking about me, my metabolism got to be kind of slow after so many severe diets. After my last competition that I have mentioned, I decided to have a child. During my pregnancy I had been eating any type of food that I was craving for. After I gave birth I had some fat and soft tissue on top, like any other new mother. It is interesting, but this pregnancy process regulated my metabolism. Four months later I was back to my normal size. Moreover, I looked even better and my metabolism increased. I could eat any type of food again and I did not get fat easy. Actually, when I wanted to eat more at one time, I felt sick. Great news! That was a sign that my stomach shrunk. But, my muscles and strength were gone, too. Even if I took it from the beginning with building the muscle mass, the muscle separations soon became more significant with more details as in the past. I noticed my muscles got more mature along with the pregnancy process. I believe other female competitors experimented the same muscle enhancement after the pregnancy. This reaction of the female's body is very interesting. The women have feminine hormones mostly but still they have times in life when the testosterone level may be high. That time I felt my muscles have a much higher ability of growth and development and if I wanted to continue competing, I would have gone to a different level in my sports career. My life took another path and I decided to stop competing because of different reasons.

I cannot complain about my life. The destiny has been brought in my way people who I could learn from and have been guided my steps for a good development. Everything is possible with a lot of work, learning, will, good judgement and a little bit of craziness. I am very thankful to God who has been lining up all the experiences in my life at the right moment.

The trophies and some of the medals have a poor manufacturing style due to the cheap budget of some competitions. The competition in Las Vegas was expected to have more budget than the ones in my country, but it did not offer medals at all. I received a small trophy for the second place but no diploma or medal. The next pages are describing a few details about my competitions and relevant photos.

2005 – 4th place – Bodybuilding National Championships of Romania

2006 – 2nd place – Bodybuilding National Championships of Romania

2007 – 3rd place – Hercules Trophy– bodybuilding

2008 – 3rd place – Bodybuilding National Championships of Romania

2008 – 3rd place – Hercules Trophy – bodybuilding

2008 – 3rd place – SuperKupa Szeghalom, Hungary – bodyfitness

2009 – 2nd place – Bodybuilding National Championships of Romania

2009 – 3rd place – Hercules Trophy – bodybuilding

2009 – 3rd place – Romania Cup – bodybuilding

2010 – 2nd place – America World Championship, Las Vegas – Figure

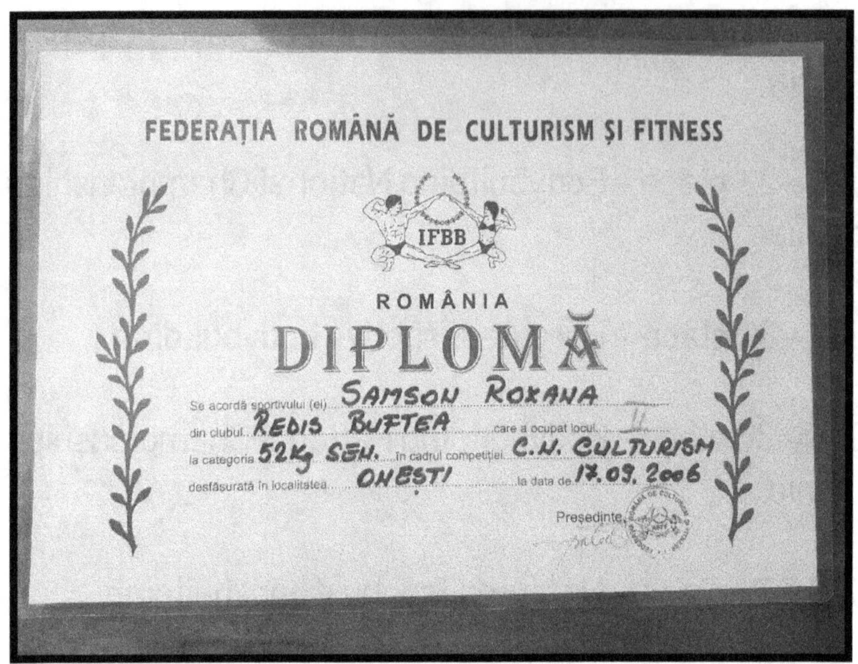

FEDERAȚIA ROMÂNĂ DE CULTURISM ȘI FITNESS
IFBB
ROMÂNIA
DIPLOMĂ
Se acordă sportivului (ei) SAMSON ROXANA
din clubul REDIS BUFTEA care a ocupat locul II
la categoria 52Kg SEN. în cadrul competiției C.N. CULTURISM
desfășurată în localitatea ONEȘTI la data de 17.09.2006
Președinte,

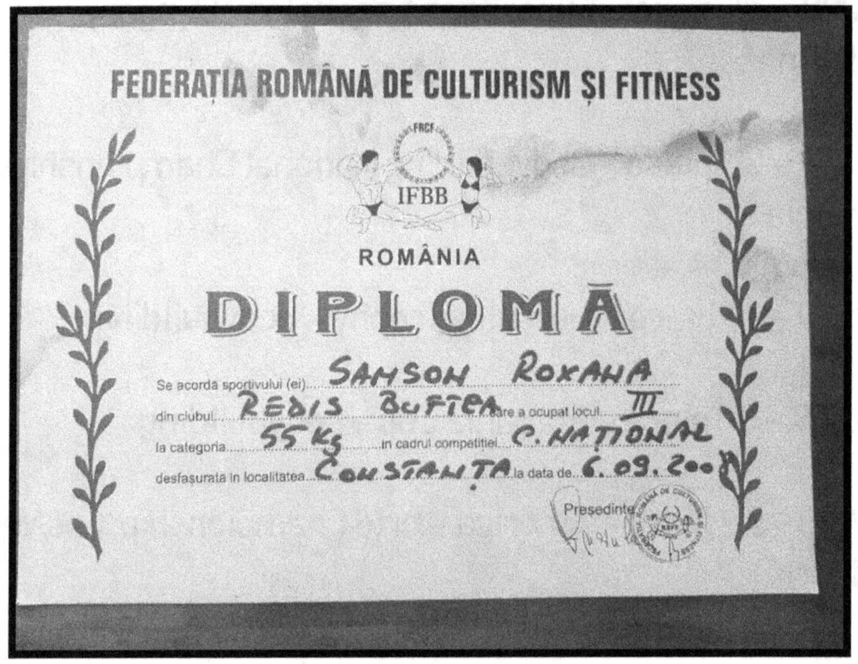

FEDERAȚIA ROMÂNĂ DE CULTURISM ȘI FITNESS
IFBB
ROMÂNIA
DIPLOMĂ
Se acorda sportivului (ei) SAMSON ROXANA
din clubul REDIS BUFTEA care a ocupat locul III
la categoria 55 Kg în cadrul competiției C. NATIONAL
desfașurata in localitatea CONSTANȚA la data de 6.09.200
Presedinte

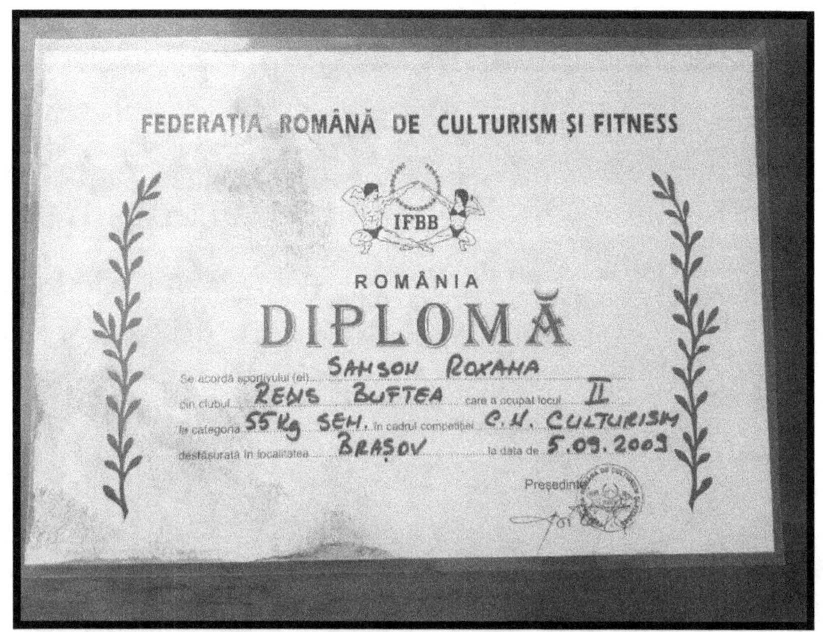

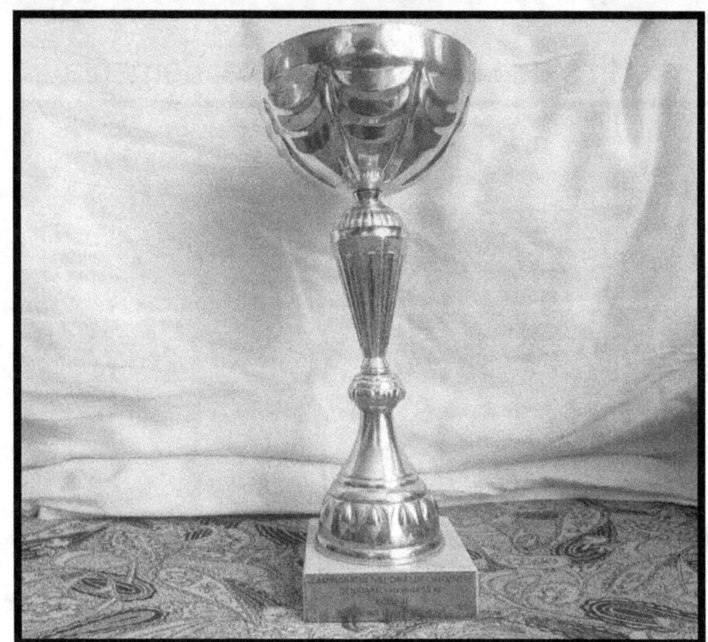

Category 55 kg, II place, 2009

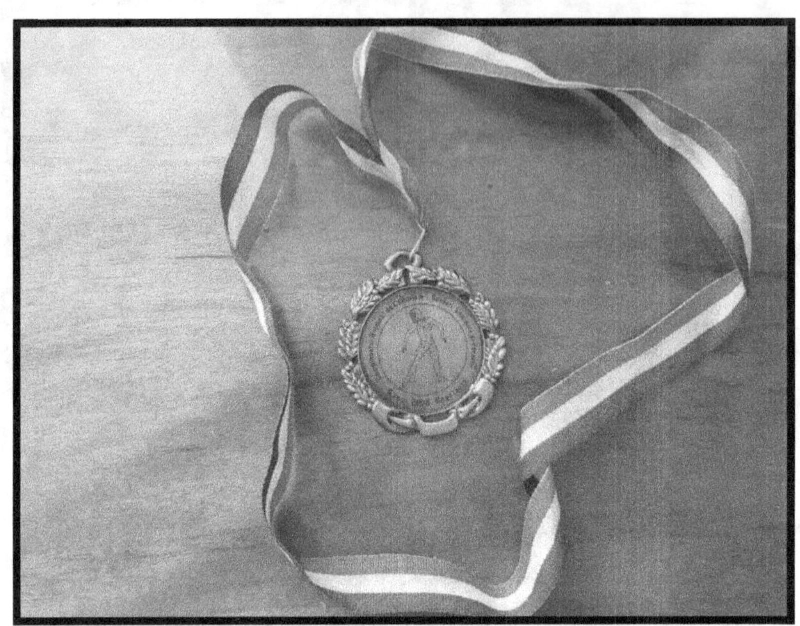

III place, 2008, Constanta, Romania

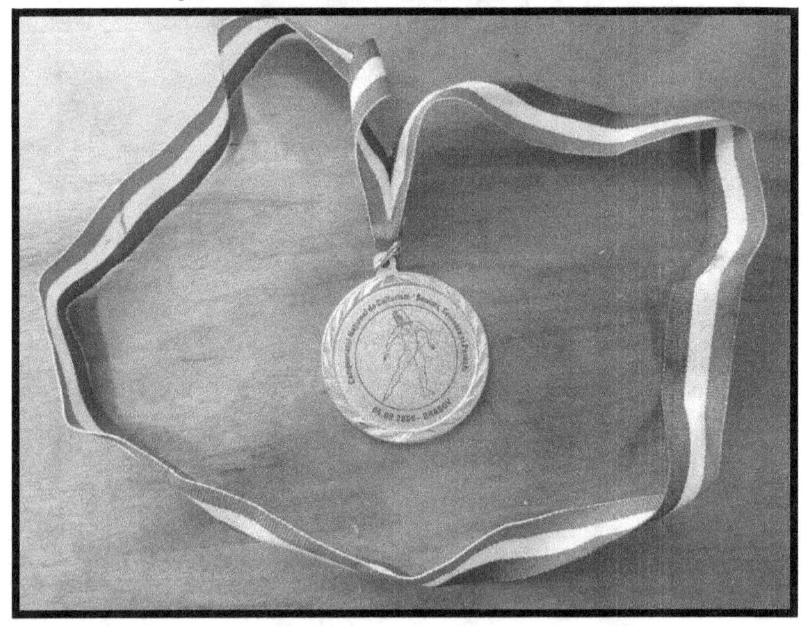

II place, 2009, Brasov, Romania

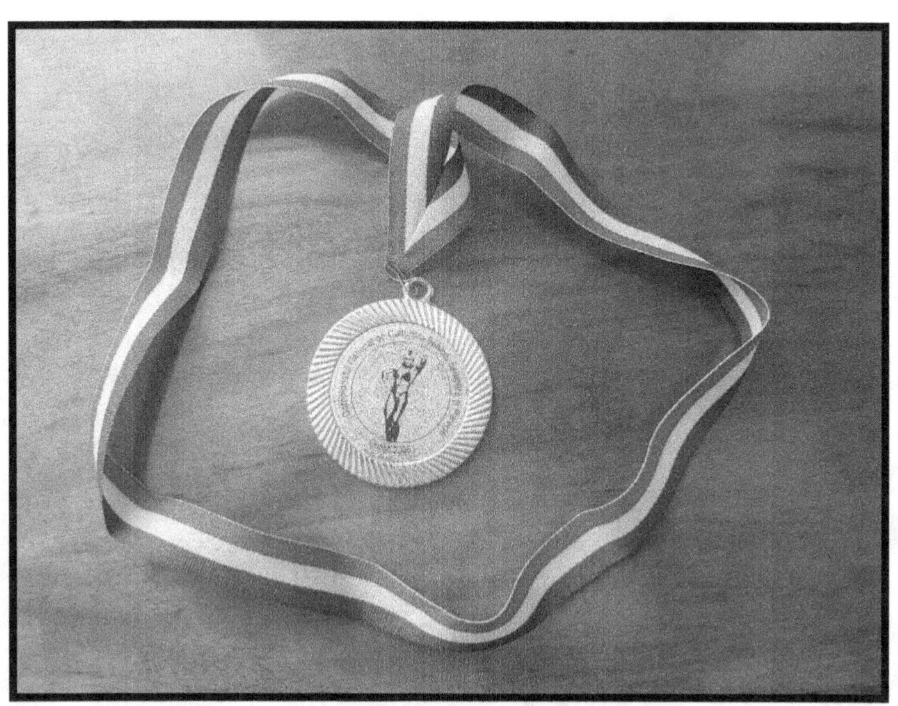

II place, 2006, Onesti, Romania

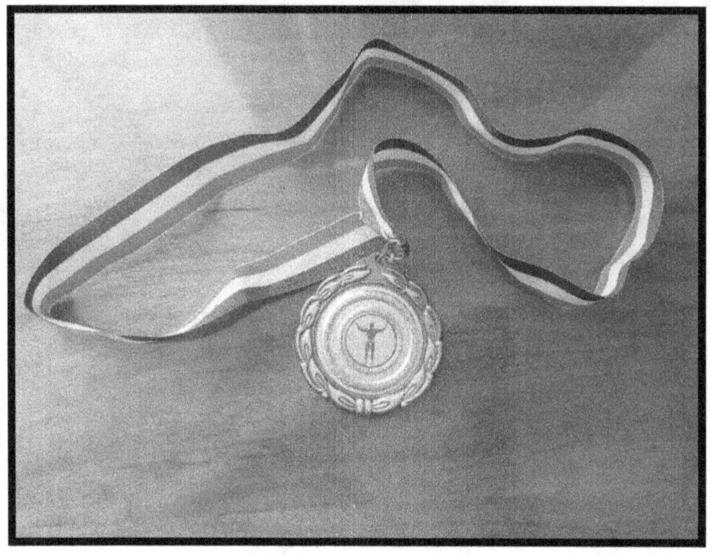

The pictures above are awards from the Romanian Bodybuilding National Championships. The following are some awards from the international competitions and the Romanian Cup.

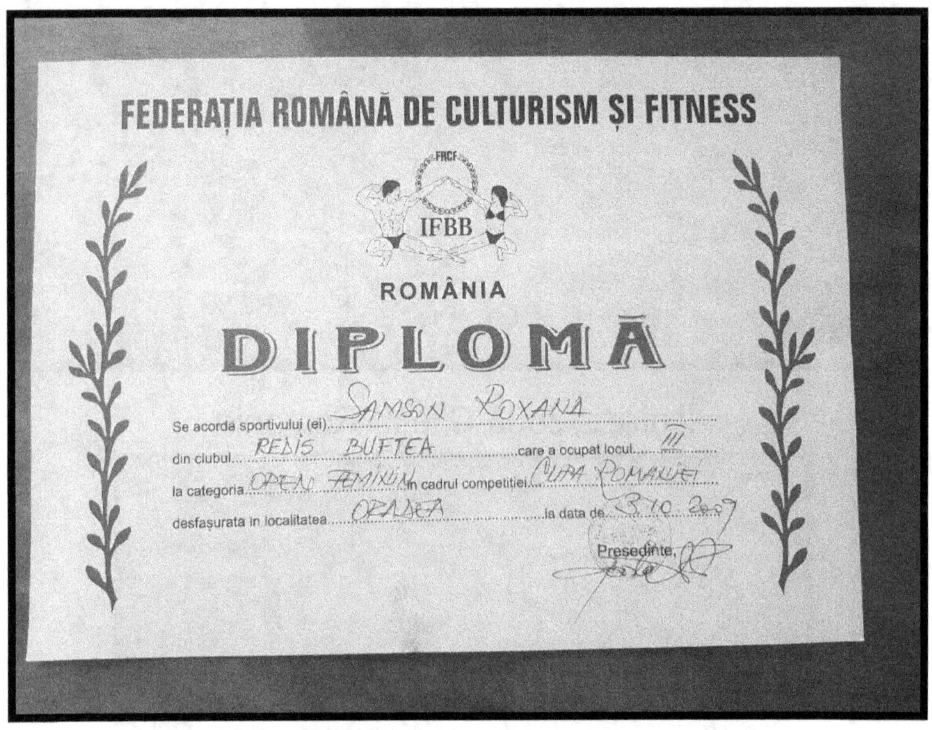

III place, Romania Cup, 2009

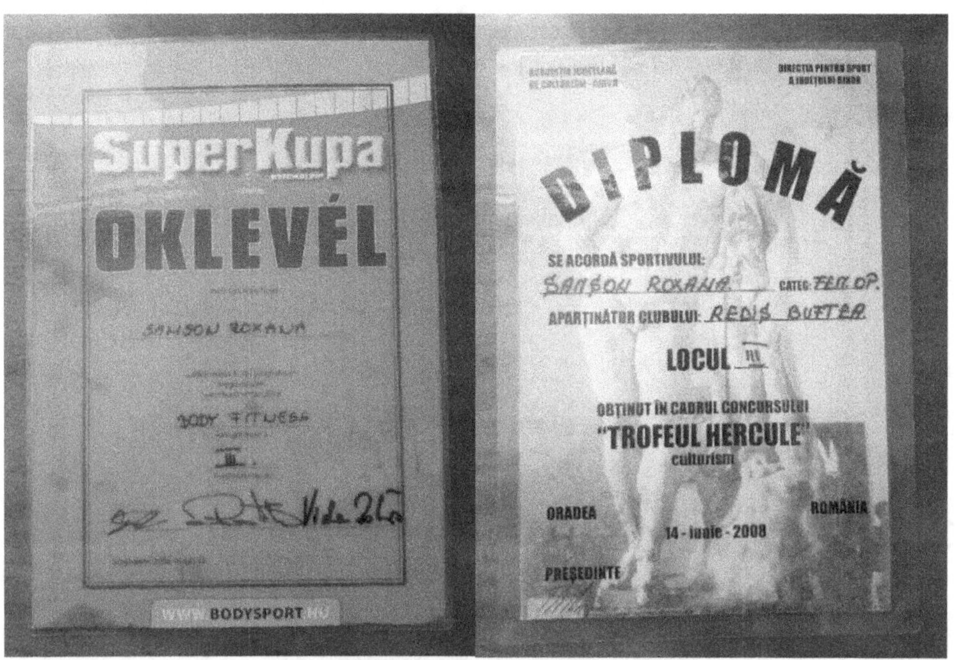

International Competitions

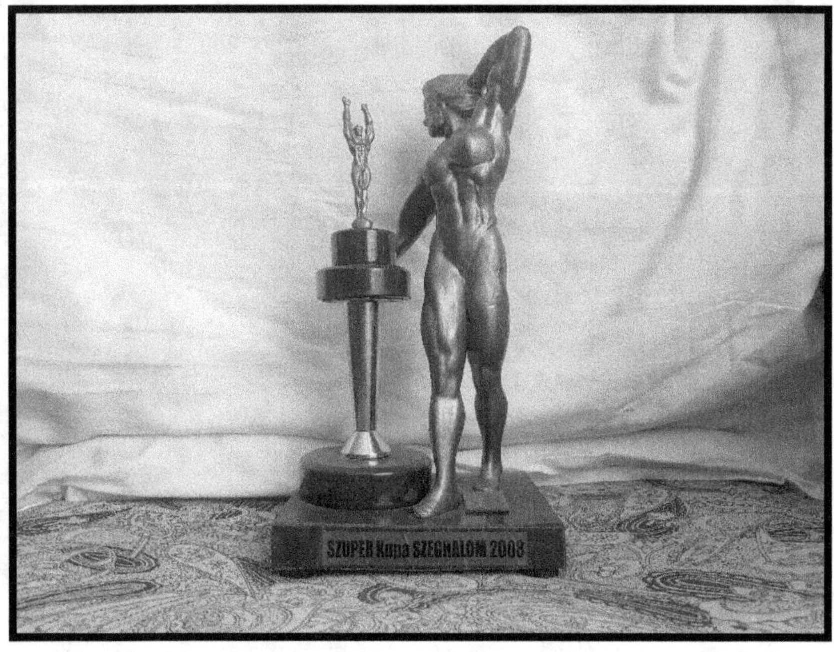

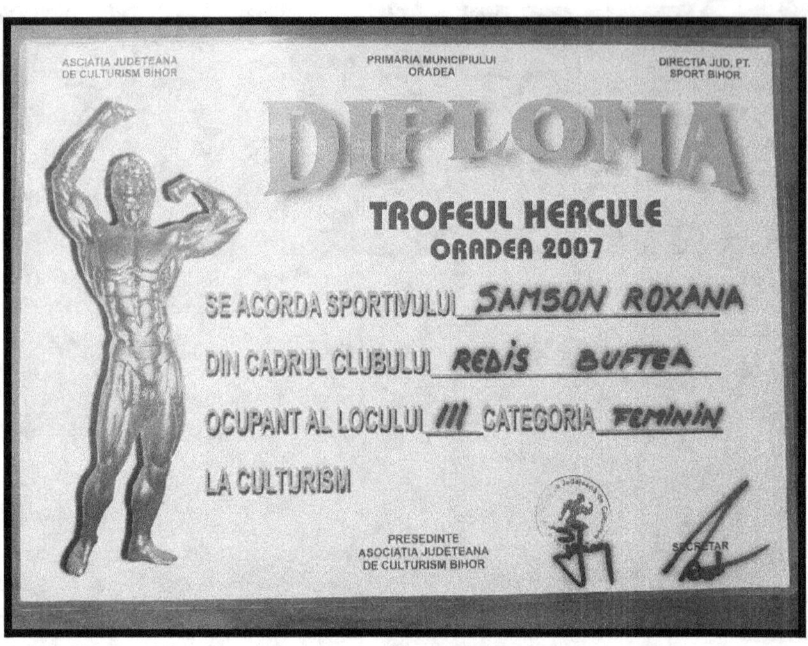
ASCIATIA JUDETEANA
DE CULTURISM BIHOR
PRIMARIA MUNICIPIULUI
ORADEA
DIRECTIA JUD. PT.
SPORT BIHOR
DIPLOMA
TROFEUL HERCULE
ORADEA 2007
SE ACORDA SPORTIVULUI SAMSON ROXANA
DIN CADRUL CLUBULUI REDIS BUFTEA
OCUPANT AL LOCULUI III CATEGORIA FEMININ
LA CULTURISM
PRESEDINTE
ASOCIATIA JUDETEANA
DE CULTURISM BIHOR
SECRETAR

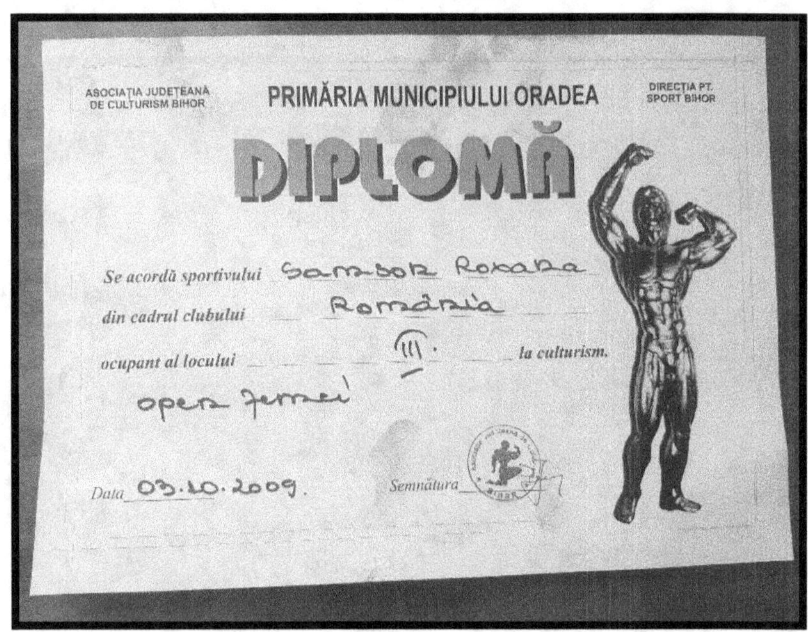
ASOCIAȚIA JUDEȚEANĂ
DE CULTURISM BIHOR
PRIMĂRIA MUNICIPIULUI ORADEA
DIRECTIA PT.
SPORT BIHOR
DIPLOMĂ
Se acordă sportivului Samson Roxana
din cadrul clubului România
ocupant al locului III la culturism.
opera femei
Data 03.10.2009. Semnătura

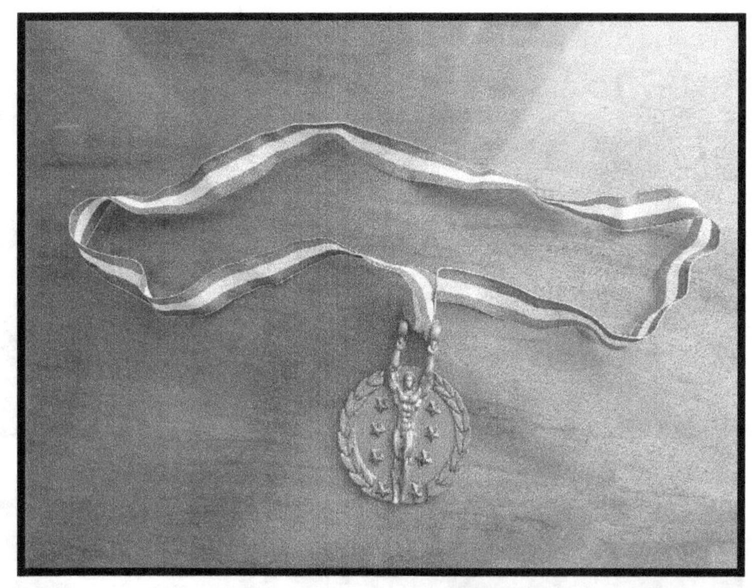

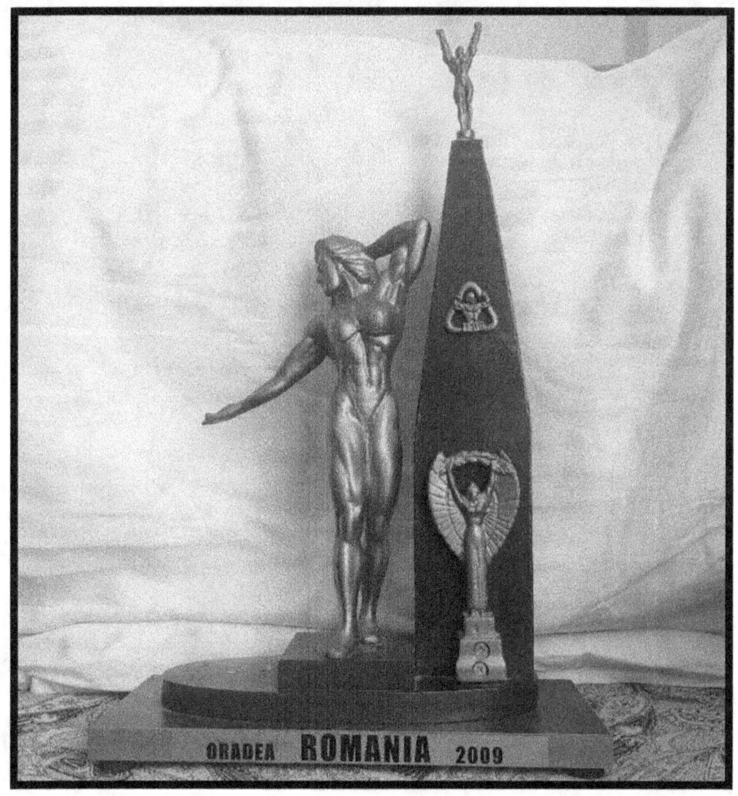

ORADEA ROMANIA 2009

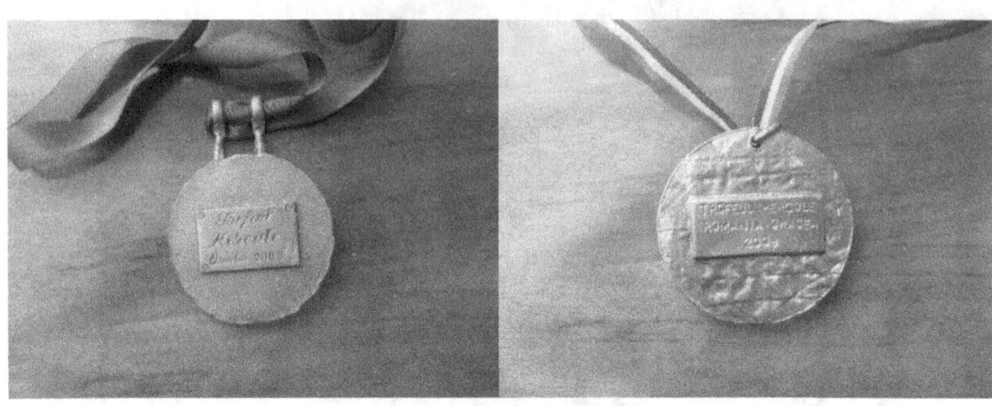

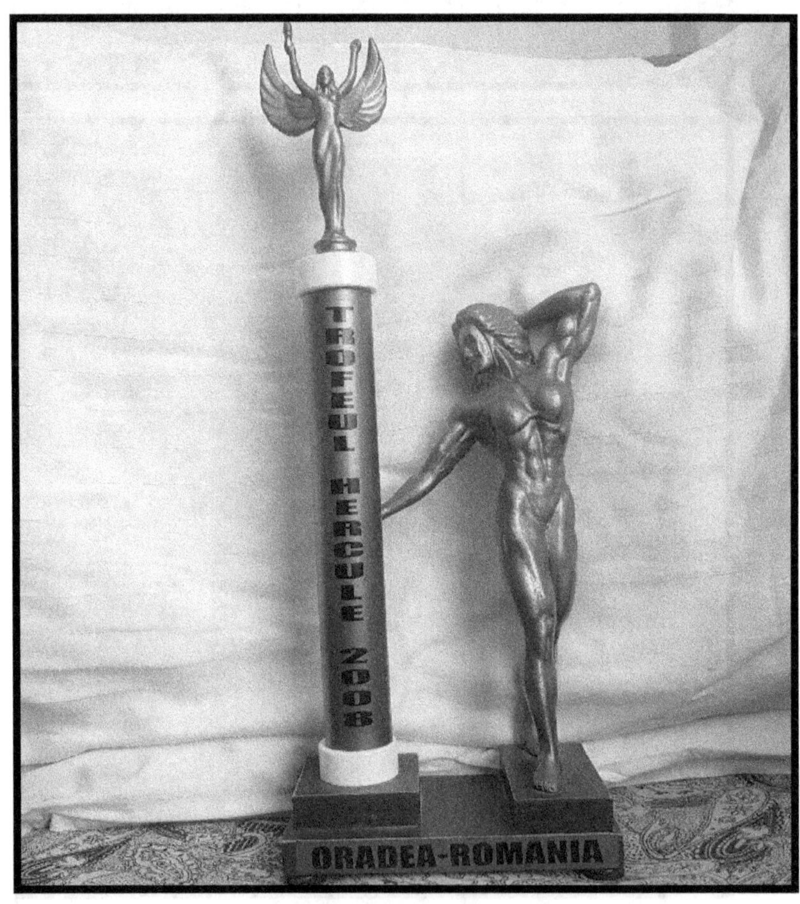

TROFEUL HERCULE
2008
ORADEA-ROMANIA

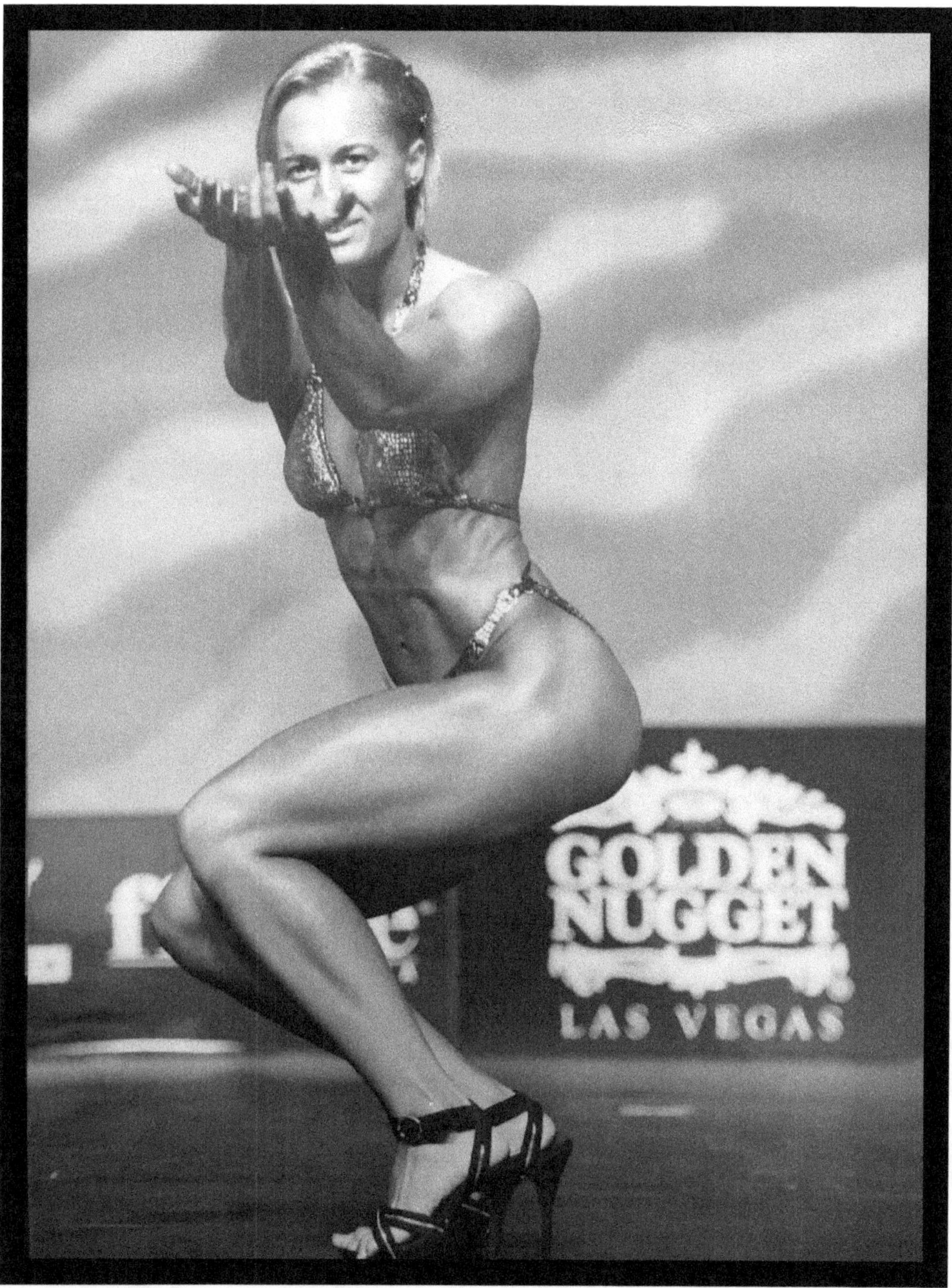

GOLDEN
NUGGET
LAS VEGAS

Roxana P. Samson